Your Guide
to Optimal Health

Your Guide to Optimal Health: Creating Your Personal Wellness Wheel

Seema Patel, MD, MPH

with Lee Kirksey, MD

Philadelphia, PA

ISBN 13: 978-0-615-22813-6

Project Credits

Project Management: Kathleen O'Hara

Copyediting: Shannon McManimon

Layout and Cover: Shannon McManimon

Write, phone, or e-mail

Dr. Seema Patel

Dr. Lee Kirksey

59 West Lancaster Avenue

Ardmore, PA 19003

phone: 610-642-2644

email: spatelmd@optimalhealthtoday.com

Web: www.optimalhealthtoday.com

To the love of my life, Lee.
Thank you for your inspiration, your faith, and your love.

Contents

PREFACE

This book is a comprehensive, step-by-step guide to help you build your Personal Wellness Wheel™. Your Personal Wellness Wheel™ is composed of eight elements needed to optimize your health and slow down your aging process. The eight elements include the most innovative, pro-active Western medical strategies, lifestyle behaviors, diet/nutrition, exercise, bio-identical hormone replacement for men and women, healthy skin, stress management, and strategies for individual success. We have integrated Eastern and Western philosophies to help you create your own individualized wellness plan.

At the end of each chapter, we provide tools to help you, the reader, build each spoke of your Personal Wellness Wheel™. These tools include interactive exercises, tests, and trend sheets to track your progress, as well as instructional sheets on nutrition, exercise, and more. The appendix provides resources for further education.

The goal of this book is to help you as an individual or a family improve your overall health and well-being. Small groups or corporations can also benefit from this individualized wellness program to improve employees' health, thereby increasing productivity and efficiency and keeping healthcare costs down. Personal health is at the center of your life and determines how you perform and how you experience your life. So begin the journey to looking good, feeling great, and living better!

Dr. Seema Patel
Dr. Lee Kirksey
Co-Founders, The Institute for Optimal Health
and Your Personal Wellness Wheel™

Tables

Quizzes, Tips, and Worksheets

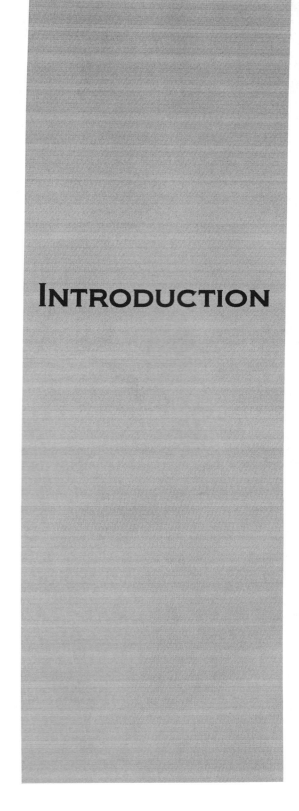

INTRODUCTION

We are what we repeatedly do.
Excellence, then, is not an act,
but a habit.

~Aristotle

If you've picked up this book, you are probably searching for a way to feel great and

live better. Many of us desire better health. In this age of the internet avalanche of options, information, and advice, how do you decide what's right for you? Maybe doctors and other health professionals have told you that everything is fine, but you don't feel quite the way you know you should or could. Maybe you've asked your doctor to help you sort through information: should I be on a low-fat, low-carb diet or a high-protein, low-carb diet? How can I lose weight? How do I minimize my chance of getting Alzheimer's or improve my energy level? Maybe you've struggled with your weight, your nutrition, dealing with stress, or the effects of growing older.

At no time during my medical training was I exposed to an integrative approach to patient care. Furthermore, I know from my years in a traditional primary care practice that the pressures of managed care do not allow for a comprehensive, holistic approach that includes patient education.

Your Guide to Optimal Health: Creating Your Personal Wellness Wheel is a comprehensive guide to help you achieve and maintain Optimal Health. Optimal Health means you perform and feel at your peak in all ways: mentally, physically, spiritually, and emotionally. In this state, you have the energy, drive, and desire to do what you want and to live the best possible life at any age. "Normal" is no longer enough; I consider "normal" the state of sitting back passively and waiting for overt changes to manifest. By the time outward change occurs, your body's dis-ease is likely well-advanced. Normal does not prevent disease or slow down the aging process. But Optimal Health is a pro-active, preventative lifestyle that can help you look good, feel great, and live better at any age.

Optimal Health is more important than ever as our population ages, healthcare costs soar, and one in two Americans have some form of chronic disease that can decrease their independence and quality of life. The traditional medical philosophy that says "don't fix it unless it is broken" is a reactive approach to disease. I have found that the best approach to preventing disease is holistic and pro-active. Our current healthcare system does not spend the time and resources to educate healthy people on how to prevent disease, but instead focuses on treating disease once it has manifested. We are then directed through a broken healthcare system full of bureaucracy and inefficiency. A fractured system in which we, the patients, become increasingly dependent on doctors. A system mired in a blinding focus on managing the acute problem. Our system is indeed broken. For the individual, family, or group who addresses this recognized healthcare deficiency with an effective, personal strategy, the rewards are significant: self-empowerment, improved health outcomes, and decreased healthcare expenses.

Optimal Health integrates the latest and most effective strategies in Western medicine with Eastern philosophy. The essence of Eastern philosophy is the interdependence and synergy of all facets of health. Eastern philosophy emphasizes creating and maintaining a balance between our inner, spiritual life and our outer, physical body; it recognizes the relationship and synergy each has with the other. When we are "balanced," we create a foundation upon which to build and experience greater states of wellness.

Being balanced requires focusing on the whole person and consistently developing and improving ourselves to achieve optimal results. Self-improvement propels us to higher levels of health and well-being, mentally, physically, spiritually and emotionally. In the East, this holistic approach addresses the various elements of health before a disease forms and can help manage a disease afterward.

In Eastern philosophy, individuals—rather than physicians—are at the center of their health. Individuals have the greatest responsibility for improving and maintaining their own health and well-being. Helping people understand that their personal health is dependent on many variables is central to treating the whole person and empowering each individual to make choices for a better, fuller life.

I have integrated this holistic approach with an Age Management and Integrated Medicine (AMIM) Program. AMIM focuses on improving our quality of life and productivity throughout life rather than simply living longer with a poor quality of life. Through working pro-actively, Age Management Medicine believes that age-related changes are true deficiencies that can be corrected. In contrast, traditional medicine believes that we must live with age-related degenerative changes. Furthermore, Age Management believes that optimal levels of health, rather than "normal" levels, are the basis of good health. As stated earlier, normal simply means that everything appears okay; it does not prevent diseases from occurring or make people feel better.

Aging is a fact of life, but *how you age* makes the difference. After the age of thirty, the aging process begins, starting a slow, steady decline in our quality of life. As we age, many of us experience weight gain along with loss of muscle mass and bone mass, physical strength, and endurance. We may have more difficulty with focus, memory, and concentration. We may experience a lower libido and other sexual dysfunctions that affect our relationships and self-esteem. We may have a lowered immune system, making us more vulnerable to illness. We can experience depression or a loss of drive, energy, passion, or vitality which affect our well-being.

Growing older is inevitable, but the quality of life that you experience in that process is highly variable. AMIM's pro-active approach to individual health can prevent disease and slow these age-related changes. AMIM can optimize your quality of life across the many years of life after age thirty. With increasing life expectancies, the ma-

THE EIGHT ELEMENTS

○ A Pro-Active Health Approach: Preventing Disease
○ The Optimal Health Lifestyle: Changing Personal Habits
○ Your Fuel for Life: Creating Ultimate Nutrition
○ The Power of Exercise: Maintaining a Youthful Mind and Body
○ Your Guide to Hormone Optimization: Restoring Your Body's Balance
○ Your Ageless Skin: Improving Your Skin at Any Age
○ Stress Management Techniques: Balancing Your Mind and Body
○ Your Strategies for Success: Choosing Your Path Wisely

jority of Americans will spend the most rewarding and memorable years of their lives after the age of 50. With AMIM, we can create a new model of healthy aging. Instead of a slow, downward decline, we can plateau, maintaining a high quality of life much longer.

To help you achieve Optimal Health and to slow the aging process, I have created a comprehensive health guide based upon your Personal Wellness Wheel™. Your Personal Wellness Wheel™ combines the latest in Western science with the holistic interdependency beliefs of Eastern philosophy. Your Personal Wellness Wheel™ is a multi-use tool that will help you develop and focus on key principles of AMIM. The Personal Wellness Wheel™ begins with you in the center, the hub of the wheel. You are the person who will change your health and overall well-being by learning to integrate the eight spokes that constantly rotate around you. These eight spokes are the key elements that will illuminate your path to Optimal Health.

As you build your Personal Wellness Wheel™ you will learn about each spoke and how to construct it. You will learn how the spokes are connected to each other and to you, as well as the unique balance that is necessary to help improve your health and well-being. This unique balance will differ from person to person.

The last part of the wheel is the rim, the outer part of the wheel that holds everything together. The rim represents the discipline needed to maintain the Personal Wellness Wheel™ and the daily need for us to be mindful of synergy and the continual need for balance among the elements.

The wheel symbolism is important for Optimal Health because it also illustrates what happens when one of the elements breaks down, if you are not at the center, or if you are not disciplined and mindful of your actions. If this occurs the wheel cannot turn; growth and self-improvement do not occur. In fact, the wheel begins to break down, and you do not feel well. If the wheel does not get repaired in a timely manner, it can lead to illness, disease, and age-related problems. This book is your guide to keeping your Personal Wellness Wheel™ balanced and always turning toward Optimal

Health.

In this journey you will learn many things. Most importantly, I would like this program to represent a tool that becomes your primary guide in your journey to Optimal Health. At the end of each chapter you will find tips on how to build each spoke of the wheel. An appendix of further resources to assist you is located at the end of the book; a more extensive, frequently updated appendix is located online at www.optimalhealthtoday.com. I firmly believe that each of you can achieve Optimal Health and maintain it. So let's begin the journey!

To looking good, feeling great, and living better always!
Seema M. Patel, MD, MPH
Lee Kirksey, MD

6 YOUR PERSONAL WELLNESS WHEEL

A PRO-ACTIVE HEALTH APPROACH: PREVENTING DISEASE

The doctor of the future will give no medication, but will interest his patients in the care of the human frame, diet and in the cause and prevention of disease.

~Thomas Edison

CONTENTS:
* common chronic diseases,
Lee Kirksey, MD
* preventative medicine
* optimal lab values
from your blood work
* building spoke one

In Aruyveda, India's traditional, natural system of medicine practiced for more than 5000 years, balance

between the mind and body comes from small, simple changes done daily in how we live, eat, think, and be, changes that promote health and well-being. The journey to Optimal Health starts with a series of small steps, beginning with understanding the creation of disease. This chapter outlines the most common chronic diseases that afflict Americans, covers the preventative measures needed for a healthy lifestyle, and then reviews laboratory results that will help you achieve Optimal Health.

In this chapter, you will learn about the following:

- ○ Common Chronic Diseases *(written by Lee Kirksey, MD)*
- ○ Preventative Medicine
- ○ Optimal Lab Values from Your Blood Work

COMMON CHRONIC DISEASES
written by Lee Kirksey, MD

In the United States, the most common cause of chronic disease and death is cardiovascular disease (CVD), followed by lung, breast, prostate, and colon cancers. Chances are that we all know of someone affected by CVD or some form of cancer. As we set the stage for collaborating with you in your journey to Optimal Health, it is important to briefly describe the process of chronic disease development. These are complex topics; each can easily require several large books to explain in detail. Yet an understanding of this chapter is an essential component of your success. Without a basic understanding of the detriments of chronic disease—a process we hope to avoid—compelling motivation to change your behaviors may be insufficient. If we want to affect sustainable behavioral changes, we must be clear about what we wish to avoid (chronic illness), just as much as we seek clarity about the ideal strategies to reach your goal of Optimal Health.

The most common cause of chronic disease and death, CVD, is relatively straightforward to discuss. The causative behaviors that contribute to the development and evolution of CVD are much clearer than those of cancer. The understanding of cancer and the complex interaction between environmental cues and genetic predisposition continues to evolve. Studies looking at genetic predisposition as well as environmental carcinogens seek to identify which factor is more directly responsible for a given cancer type.

I give an example to patients who are interested in understanding more about causation and potential prevention of disease. Questions usually arise when patients who have seen an immediate family member suffer a challenging medical condition such as a heart attack or stroke inquire about their own risk factors. My sense is that they are actually asking, "How much control do I have over my medical condition? Has the damage that I have already done irreversibly injured my body, or can I make changes now that will turn things around?"

I respond this way: I classify our population into three groups only for the purpose of discussing the complex interaction between environment and genetics in disease causation. The first group is the child, adolescent, or young adult who develops, very early in life, some autoimmune or malignant cancer like a breast cancer. In general, one of two things likely occurred. The person was either born with some abnormal gene that expressed this cancer at a young age or some gene mutation occurred relatively early in this individual's life. Regardless of how this person lived or the environmental insults that occurred, he or she probably had a predisposition in the form of an abnormal cell line at birth or a mutation (change) that occurred early in life to a vulnerable gene. To some extent, this group of people is genetically vulnerable or just darn unlucky. This is the group most profoundly affected by periodic scientific discoveries that identify on the gene map the location of changes associated with these illnesses.

On the other end of the spectrum are the people interviewed on a news program because of their 90th birthday celebrations. Cognitively, they appear to perform very well, they are quite active, and they lament the changes they have seen over their near-century of life. When inevitably asked about what they believe to be their secret for longevity, they respond that there is no secret; they have lived "regular lives" with no significant attention to healthy behavior. Listening to their stories, it becomes very evident that these people have done nothing special to add years to their lives and sometimes, quite the contrary. My grandfather is the perfect example of this individual. As he approaches his 91st birthday, he doesn't hesitate to tell you that he smoked until he was 73. Much of his life was spent as a bricklayer, inhaling what to me are lung pollutants. He never ate any special diet. Aside from the broken hip that sidelined him at age 85, he can't remember the last time he was ill.

Such a person is genetically resistant to disease. For unidentified reasons, no environmental stimulus was able to disrupt the complex cycle of cell growth to any significant degree; cancer infection and cardiovascular disease were held at bay. This group is clearly a small percentage of our population.

By and large, most of our population will fall within the third group, the bell curve of the descriptive spectrum of disease. We are not born with any major genetic abnormalities which affect our health early in life. Over the course of life, our body is exposed to various environmental factors, some outside of our control (food toxins, secondhand smoke) and some because of lifestyle choices that we make (sun exposure, excessive saturated fat intake, lack of exercise, stress, and the list goes on). Ultimately, some environmental stimulus like cigarette smoking or chronic inflammation will cause some gene to mutate. If the gene is repaired, nothing happens. If it causes rapid, uncontrolled cellular proliferation, perhaps we will develop a chronic illness or a type of cancer. I use this example to suggest that the vast majority of our population has a significant component of our personal health under our own control. If we can limit environmental insults and improve our body's ability to repair them when they inevitably occur, then we really do have the best opportunity to live a healthy life.

Throughout the Optimal Health program, we refer to "balance," a state of equilibrium within our bodies and between ourselves and our environment. The importance of balance is demonstrated by the body's immune function. The immune system performs a dual purpose: It is the body's barrier to environmental insults, and it effectively manages internal uprising. It is the defense against bacterial or viral infection, and it oversees the millions of cell divisions that occur over the course of our lifetimes. As with many of the silent bodily functions that occur automatically without our knowledge, twenty-four hours a day and seven days a week, it's quite amazing in its capacity.

PREVENTING CANCER

The development of cancer is a result of altered immune function. Not many other medical terms provoke the same emotional reaction as cancer, the "Big C." In fact, the term has such a uniformly accepted negative connotation that most people don't ask what type of cancer. They just accept that it's cancer and that all cancers are bad. "Aunt Sallie has cancer." Not early cancer or late cancer . . . just cancer. Furthermore, most people are uncertain as to what actually causes cancer. And it's not difficult to see why. Each day brings new information about another "association" between a chemical or an environmental agent and cancer development. One week, a cup of coffee is associated with a decreased incidence of cancer. The next week, three cups of coffee is associated with an increased chance of cancer. It's utterly confusing to the most conscientious and well-read lay-person, and I admit that as a physician, it's equally frustrating.

This uncertainty about what causes cancer and the preventative measures to avoid it is, in my opinion, at the heart of what people fear most about the disease: "How can I protect myself from a disease when I don't understood where it comes from?" If I know what causes a disease and still eat foods or commit behaviors that might lead to the disease, some unstated thought seems to suggest that while tragic, the illness can be explained. Lung cancer in a long-term smoker is a good example of this mindset. We hope that by describing the fundamental role of the immune system and its contribution to the development of cancer, you will feel empowered to optimize your body's defense.

An attempt to understand the genesis of cancer must begin with a description of the immune system and its function. Stated simply, cancer is caused by malfunction of the immune system. Two basic mechanisms of failure exist within the immune system. First, the immune cells that protect against infection or early cell damage can fail to recognize injury to a cell and allow this process to evolve in an unregulated fashion. Second, immune cells can turn against the normal tissues that are being protected and begin to harm the body. This is what happens when a person suffers from an autoimmune process like arthritis, allergies, or chronic, low-grade inflammation.

Why does the immune system need to "police" abnormal cells? Over the course of our lifetimes, the cells of our body undergo trillions of divisions. When a cell divides, the DNA–the special code for proteins that determines our cells' composition–is replicated. During this replication process, the sequence of DNA code may be disrupted by reversing or dropping a code sequence. Several consequences may occur when an abnormal coding sequence is created. The incorrectly coded cell may die; it may be recognized as incorrect and destroyed; it may continue to survive inactive and inconsequential; or it may go on to proliferate in an unchecked fashion. The last option may lead to the development of abnormal tissue. Over the course of our lives, these cell changes (mutations) happen many times. Fortunately in most cases, it is a benign occurrence with no detrimental consequences. In a person with a competent and vigilant immune system, the chances are greater that abnormal cells will be detected and destroyed.

Several events happen over time that may influence cell reproduction. As we grow older, the number of cell mutations accumulates. This is partly a natural function of time and would occur in the absence of outside factors. Our lifestyle choices and personal behaviors also have a profound impact on how frequently and how severely our cells are insulted. As we will learn in later chapters, factors such as a low-fiber diet, a lack of exercise, and chronic stress each act in their own way to impact cell function.

Additionally, as we grow older, our immune systems may begin to deteriorate, contributing to the imbalance of accumulating abnormal cells. This increase in abnormal cells theoretically increases the chance of cancer as we age.

As stated earlier, our goal in Optimal Health is to create a step-wise program to improve your personal health. Equally important in this process are behaviors to avoid, including those that have been shown to increase the development of various forms of cancer. The reoccurring, fundamental theme of our Optimal Health Program is that an ounce of prevention is worth a pound of cure. A sound personal wellness strategy prevents chronic disease from developing through:

- ❖ Appropriately using available screening measures for early detection of cancer and CVD
- ❖ Avoiding environmental triggers for cancer and CVD

❖ Implementing nutrition, exercise, hormonal, and stress management strategies that optimize your body's immune defense.

Tremendous amounts of governmental and private-sector funding have been directed to cancer research. The Susan G. Komen Foundation is a perfect example of the impact of a successful public awareness campaign. I would venture to guess that most of us have donated money or time to a breast cancer event. I look at the Komen Foundation as one of the bellwether standards for health awareness campaigns. The major focus of all awareness campaigns is early detection—and for a good reason.

Identifying cancers early, when they are small and have not spread outside the area of local formation, allows for the most successful treatment. Because there are many types of cancer which may behave differently, it's hard to discuss cancers in general terms. Some are more resistant to surgical excision, radiation, or chemotherapy. But in general, if a tumor is completely surgically excised (with no residual lymph nodes), there is a 30-40 percent chance that it will return. If the cancer has spread beyond its original area at the time of detection, a patient may undergo surgical excision followed by chemotherapy and radiation. In this case, the chance of recurrence is about 70-80 percent. Again, I reluctantly present these general statistics (realizing that a topic like cancer prognosis is difficult to generalize) to illustrate that prevention is a much better strategy. Most oncology literature suggests that survival for major cancers has improved very slowly over time, despite the diligent research efforts occurring in oncology.

Because of the complexity of this immune process, regulating its performance is not as straightforward as managing the prevention of CVD. We can create a comprehensive program for you that, in the absence of some profound genetic predisposition to CVD, will result in a low likelihood of developing severe CVD. Because the contributions of environment and genetics are less clear with cancer, the blueprint is valuable but less certain. I am certain that prevention is much more reliable than treatment with regard to cancer.

If we hope to diminish our risk of cancer, we must first look closely at our environment for clues on risk reduction. Up to 40 percent of all cancers are related to tobacco use. Another 30 percent of cancers are related to the food we consume and our gastrointestinal tract (including stomach and colon cancers). For instance, various dietary factors including low fiber and high saturated fat and inflammatory bowel conditions have been associated with cancers of the stomach and colon. And excessive alcohol intake is associated with cancer of the liver and esophagus. Overweight individuals are at higher risk for breast cancer and prostate cancer, probably because many of the sex hormones that regulate these cancers are sequestered in fat.

We can see these factors in the tables that follow. Table 1 on the next page describes the leading causes of death in the United States in 2000. The number of people dying as a result of cardiovascular disease (CVD) far exceeds the number of Americans who die from the next five causes. Table 2 lists the lifestyle behaviors that are actually responsible for the medical illnesses.

TABLE 1. LEADING CAUSES OF DEATH IN THE UNITED STATES IN 2000*

Cause of Death	Number of Deaths	Death Rate per 100,000 Population
Heart disease	710,760	258.2
Malignant neoplasm	553,091	200.9
Cerebrovascular disease	167,661	60.9
Chronic lower respiratory tract disease	122,009	44.3
Unintentional injuries	97,900	35.6
Diabetes mellitus	69,301	25.2
Influenza and pneumonia	65,313	23.7
Alzheimer's disease	49,558	18.0
Nephritis, nephrotic syndrome, & nephrosis	37,251	13.5
Septicemia	31,224	11.3
Other	499,283	181.4
Total	**2,403,351**	**873.1**

TABLE 2. ACTUAL CAUSES OF DEATH IN THE UNITED STATES, 1990 & 2000

Actual Cause	Number (%) in 1990**	Number (%) in 2000**
Tobacco	400,000 (19%)	435,000 (18.1%)
Poor diet and physical inactivity	300,000 (14%)	400,000 (16.6%)
Alcohol consumption	100,000 (5%)	85,000 (3.5%)
Microbial agents	90,000 (4%)	75,000 (3.1%)
Toxic agents	60,000 (3%)	55,000 (2.3%)
Motor vehicle	25,000 (1%)	43,000 (1.8%)
Firearms	35,000 (2%)	29,000 (1.2%)
Sexual behavior	30,000 (1%)	20,000 (0.8%)
Illicit drug use	20,000 (<1%)	17,000 (0.7%)
Total	**1,060,000 (50%)**	**1,159,000 (48.2%)**

*Data from CDC, 2007. **The percentages are for all deaths.*

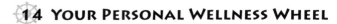

The second cancer avoidance strategy is improving our immune function. Remember that earlier I referred to mutations that inevitably occur over our lives. Millions of cells will divide, die, and be replaced. Ideally, if we can increase the efficiency at which damaged cells are identified and disposed of, increase the accuracy of new cell creation, and eliminate environmental stimuli which may damage cells, we theoretically decrease our chances of cancer over our lifetimes.

Let's look at an example. Sun exposure is a perfect example of a behavior that when performed in moderation is healthy, but when performed in excess may lead to a deadly skin cancer. Sun exposure is beneficial to our bodies because it facilitates the production of Vitamin D. Vitamin D is beneficial to our cardiovascular and immune health. Sun exposure also stimulates brain centers that are responsible for mood elevation. In fact, it's very common for people to feel a decrease in energy during the winter months when sun exposure may be limited. However, in excess, sun exposure can be quite harmful, causing damage to the very proteins that make up the cells in the skin. This damage may result in various forms of skin cancer. Those at greatest risk for skin cancer appear to be fair-skinned, those who have suffered severe sunburns, and those who have a family history of skin cancer. Prevention is aimed at limiting sun exposure to fifteen to twenty minutes daily. All sun exposure should be mitigated by the use of sunblocks.

Using sun exposure as an example of factors on the environmental level, decreasing our exposure to the harmful effects of radiation from the sun is a reliable way of decreasing our chance of skin cancer. On the immune system level, using a supplement system to replace antioxidants, also known as free radical scavengers, helps to repair damaged cells ("free radical" refers to a damaged cell type). Finally, improving our ability to successfully manage stress is crucial to maintaining a strong and competent immune system.

Preventing Cardiovascular Disease (CVD)

Of the chronic medical conditions, none is more pervasive and destructive to individual health than cardiovascular disease (CVD). Our hope is that our partnership with you through this book and our online program will provide you with the education and applied understanding to prevent CVD through the creation and maintenance of a sound and disciplined personal health program. With one in two Americans dying from CVD, most families will be affected in some way by this illness. We would be remiss if we did not describe the "silent killer" in a way that allows you to understand the prevention, identification, treatment, and emotional consequences of this common chronic disease process.

Several medical disorders may contribute to the development of CVD. These are best categorized into two categories: non-modifiable and modifiable.

Non-Modifiable	_Modifiable_
❖ Hypertension	❖ Smoking
❖ Diabetes	❖ Being Overweight
❖ High Cholesterol	❖ Diet/Nutrition
❖ "Bad Genes"	❖ Physical Inactivity

Being overweight, which 60 percent of Americans are, is a precursor to many medical conditions, including hypertension, diabetes, and high cholesterol. If we believe that high blood pressure, diabetes, and high cholesterol are largely a result of what we eat, then our genetics are the only non-modifiable factor. As one commercial proudly states, it all boils down to "food or family." The condition of your blood vessels is a consequence of (1) what you put in your body (fatty foods, high sugar content, and nicotine), (2) the familial genetic traits that were passed on to you, or (3) poor lifestyle choices such as smoking.

All of the medical conditions which lead to CVD are directly affected by a lifetime of our eating habits and our family genetics or some combination of these two factors. But how do lifestyle behaviors create CVD? What causes blockages in the blood vessels of the human body?

Blockages develop when repetitive injury to the blood vessel lining occurs over time. The body responds to this localized ulceration or plaque by "patching" the area with platelets (plugs) and clotting factors; the damaged area eventually forms a "scar." When this occurs repetitively, the lumen (opening) of the blood vessel narrows. This decreases the amount of oxygen and nutrients that may pass through the blood vessel to supply the ultimate destination (such as the brain or the heart). If a high-grade narrowing already exists and this scar (atherosclerotic plaque) erupts, then the immediate "patching" process may cause the blood vessel to close off completely. This usually leads to a myocardial infarction (heart attack) or cerebral infarction (stroke). This is why anti-platelet medications like aspirin may decrease the risk of heart attack or stroke.

The agents that cause these repetitive injuries to blood vessels are:
- ❖ High blood cholesterol levels
- ❖ High dietary cholesterol intake
- ❖ High blood glucose (sugar) levels
- ❖ Hypertension
- ❖ Nicotine.

Blood Cholesterol and Dietary Cholesterol

I intentionally distinguish high levels of dietary cholesterol from high levels of blood cholesterol. Doctors Joseph Goldstein and Michael Brown won the Nobel Prize in Medicine in 1985 for the discovery of LDL cholesterol receptors. There are two subtypes of cholesterol: LDL (remember this by associating L with lousy) and HDL (H for happy). It is possible that if I have a high dietary cholesterol intake–two sausages, three eggs, and buttered toast for breakfast–my blood cholesterol level will remain essentially unchanged because I have a high number of cholesterol receptors. Cholesterol receptors, located in the liver, bind and remove cholesterol from your bloodstream. The more cholesterol receptors you have, the more efficiently you remove cholesterol from the bloodstream. The fewer cholesterol receptors you have, the greater the likelihood that your cholesterol will increase when you eat dietary cholesterol. The number of cholesterol receptors that you have is, to a great degree, genetically determined.

High Blood Pressure

Over time, the force of elevated blood pressure traumatizes the arterial wall and injures the blood vessel lining. In response to this type of injury, the repetitive cycle of healing occurs, and scar tissue accumulates. This creates a vicious cycle. As the vessel becomes increasingly blocked and rigid from scar tissue development, the blood pressure increases within the vessel. The increased blood pressure creates more injury and so forth.

In other circumstances, elevated blood pressure disrupts the integrity of the cells of the blood vessel. In other words, the blood pressure is high enough that blood leaks outside the blood vessel into the tissues, causing injury. This may occur in the brain, leading to a bleeding (hemorrhagic) stroke as compared to a lack of oxygen (ischemic or infarct) injury.

Nicotine

Nicotine is one of the most immediately correctable causes of CVD. Most people recognize the association between smoking and lung cancer, but the association between CVD and smoking is just as direct, and smoking is probably responsible for more CVD-related deaths. Nicotine is inhaled and filtered by the lungs. It is then absorbed into the bloodstream where the blood nicotine levels cause injury to the lining of the blood vessels. There is evidence that these nicotine levels contribute to the low-grade, indolent inflammatory process that is the hallmark of systemic degeneration in adults associated with skin changes and cancer development.

Diet/Nutrition

The World Health Organization (WHO) has coined the term "globesity," referring to the problem of global obesity and the looming public healthcare crisis caused by excessive weight gain. The WHO suggests that obesity is approaching smoking as a risky lifestyle choice and its potentially deleterious impact on world health.

Although a complete discussion of nutritional strategies is beyond the scope of this book, Chapter Three provides a detailed description of sound, evidence-based dietary principles. If we focus on the major culprit that affects CVD, community-based programs that emphasize decreasing the incidence of obesity will have the highest return on our educational and financial investment, particularly if these programs are partially focused on developing positive dietary habits in children and decreasing our adolescents' "video-game" culture of sedentary lifestyles.

TEST YOUR KNOWLEDGE OF PHYSICAL ACTIVITY & HEART DISEASE

Questions 1-8 are true/false.

1. Regular physical activity can reduce your chances of getting heart disease.
2. Most people get enough physical activity from their normal daily routines.
3. You don't have to train like a marathon runner to become more physically fit.
4. People who need to lose weight are the only ones who benefit from regular exercise.
5. All exercises give you the same benefits.
6. The older you are, the less active you need to be.
7. The most common risk in exercising is injury to the muscles and joints.
8. You should consult a doctor before starting a physical activity program.
9. Eliminating heart disease would increase U.S. life expectancy by how many years?
10. How many women die of heart disease in the United States? 1 every 1, 5, 7, or 9 minutes

ANSWERS

1. True. Regular physical activity decreases your risk of developing cardiovascular disease. Sedentary individuals have twice the risk of developing CVD.
2. False. More than half of Americans get no exercise outside of work. Americans are "busy but not active." Current recommendations are for low to moderate intensity exercise at least five days, if not each day, of the week. This may include brisk walking.
3. True. The key is to get started. If you exercise "occasionally," work it into each day of the week. To get started, exercise at lunch or with a friend at the end of the day.
4. False. Everyone benefits from exercise. It increases muscle tone, burns off excess calories, and improves blood pressure and cholesterol levels.
5. False. Different age groups benefit from different exercises. Aerobic exercise refers to brisk walking or other activities. Exercises like tai chi can increase flexibility and balance.
6. False. Exercise is critical to slowing aging. Medical literature shows that consistent exercise improves quality of life and decreases the risk of Alzheimer's.
7. True. Exercise-related injuries are most commonly due to muscle strains and may be minimized by appropriate stretching and "listening" to your body.
8. True. If over age 40, ask your physician about a cardiac stress test prior to beginning exercise.
9. The average life expectancy of people born in the United States is now 77.3 years. But if all major forms of cardiovascular disease—such as stroke, heart attack, and high blood pressure—were done away with, the average person would gain about seven additional years of life. A heart attack can shorten your life by nearly twelve years.
10. Every minute a woman dies of cardiovascular disease. Yet most women still believe their Number 1 health threat is cancer and that heart disease is a "man's disease." More women than men die of cardiovascular disease (including stroke). Women often don't recognize when they're having a heart attack because they aren't familiar with the symptoms of a heart attack in women.

PREVENTATIVE MEDICINE

In your quest to prevent disease, getting the recommended tests in this section begins your journey to Optimal Health.

Pap smears: For Optimal Health, I recommend that women do this annually for the detection of cervical cancer. If you have had an abnormality, you need to follow up as indicated by your physician.

Mammography: For Optimal Health, annual screening begins at age 40. If you have a close relative with breast cancer (mother, grandmother, sister) who was diagnosed under age 50, you need to have your first mammogram ten years before her age at diagnosis and then annually or as your doctor recommends. Speak with your doctor about a breast MRI which provides a better technique for identifying early breast cancer if you are at risk.

Colonoscopy: Screening begins at age 50 and then as recommended by your physician. If you have a family history of colon cancer, hereditary colorectal syndromes, polyps, inflammatory bowel disease, and/or symptoms of blood in the stools, chronic constipation, or diarrhea, speak with your physician about screening because you may be at higher risk.

Vaccinations: Please discuss with your physician the need for vaccinations as well as any contraindications.

❑ Tetanus: Everyone should update this every ten years or every five years if you get cut.

❑ Hepatitis B: Is for high-risk individuals such as healthcare workers, patients with liver disease, and people who travel extensively. The series of three vaccinations should last a lifetime if you respond to them.

❑ Hepatitis A: Is for patients with liver disease and for people who are traveling to developing countries.

❑ Flu vaccine: Is recommended for those over age 65, under age 2, healthcare workers, residents of nursing homes, people with chronic diseases such as heart disease, diabetes, and for any healthy person who wants it. The vaccine is directed at the most common flu strains of the year. If you do get the flu, your symptoms will be milder. If you get another strain, you will have no protection.

❑ Pneumonia vaccine: The adult pneumococcal vaccine is recommended for all people over age 65. For those who have had any chronic illness such as heart disease, diabetes, lung disease, or HIV, it is recommended once before age 65 and then again after age 65.

❑ Zoster vaccine: Prevents shingles in people over 60 years of age.

❑ Other: Specific groups of adults need other vaccinations; please discuss your needs with your physician. For more information, please visit the CDC site at www.cdc.gov/vaccines/spec-grps/adults.htm

Bone density: Bone density testing measures how dense your bones are. The denser your bones, the healthier they are. The less dense they are, the greater your risk for osteoporosis and a subsequent fracture.

You can measure your bone density with either a DEXA scan or a quantitative CT scan. The dual energy X-ray absorptiometry (DEXA) scan measures the bone density at your hip or spine and is preferred for diagnosing osteoporosis. The quantitative CT (QCT) provides detailed, 3-D images and can take into account the effects of aging and diseases other than osteoporosis on your bones.

❑ T-score: Your T-score is your bone density compared with normal expectations for a healthy young adult of your sex. Your T-score is the number of units—standard deviations (SD)—that your bone density is above or below the standard.

T-score	What your score means
Above -1	Your bone density is considered normal.
Between -1 and -2.5	Your score is a sign of osteopenia, a condition in which bone density is below normal and may lead to osteoporosis.
Below -2.5	Your bone density indicates you have osteoporosis.

Optimally, everyone should have a bone density test. One out of two women and one out of four men have osteoporosis. The people at highest risk for osteoporosis are those who

❖ are postmenopausal women
❖ are small-framed Caucasian or Asian women
❖ have primary hyperparathyroidism or hyperthyroidism
❖ have been on long-term steroid therapy, such as prednisone
❖ are smokers or drink excessively
❖ have a sedentary lifestyle
❖ have decreased calcium and Vitamin D intake over a prolonged time period.

Optimal levels are a T score above (-1) for both sexes and all ethnic groups. If your score is less, your doctor will address this with you. Your options for treatment will vary depending on the score. They include Vitamin D3, calcium, hormone replacement therapy (for both men and women, if you are a candidate), and the biphosphanates (medications to help build bone mass such as Fosamax™, Boniva™, or Actonel™). Other natural ways to build bone density are good nutrition, not smoking, and exercise.

Rectal exam: For Optimal Health, annual exams begin after age 40 for both men and women. Your physician may also check your stool for blood during this time or provide you with testing material to do so at home.

Eye exam: If you wear glasses or contacts, you need an annual eye exam. If you are over age 40 or have a chronic illness that can affect your vision, you should have your eyes checked annually or as indicated by a specialist.

Dental exam: You should see your dentist annually or as recommended. You should have your teeth cleaned professionally twice per year. At home I recommend flossing, a tongue cleaner, an oral rinse, and an oscillitating toothbrush that can help decrease plaque formation and reduce the bacteria in your mouth that have been linked to heart disease. You can visit our Website at www.optimalhealthtoday.com to learn about or purchase oscillitating toothbrushes. If you grind your teeth, wear a mouth guard to protect your teeth from enamel erosion.

Full-body skin checks: Skin cancer is most common in fair-skinned people and in sun-exposed areas of the body, but all ethnic groups can get skin cancer. Everyone should have an annual full-body skin examination with a dermatologist.

Cardiac stress test: You need a cardiac stress test if
- ❖ you are over age 40 and are beginning an exercise program.
- ❖ you are having symptoms of chest pain, shortness of breath, or irregular heart rhythms.
- ❖ you have a family history of early heart disease.
- ❖ your physician recommends it.

For people who have no symptoms or history of cardiovascular disease, I recommend other imaging tests that may identify the early stages of cardiovascular disease and may permit a more aggressive approach to preventative strategies for cholesterol control, blood pressure control, and lifestyle.

❑ Carotid intimal thickening: This carotid ultrasound of the neck measures the thickness of the artery. The more thickening you have of the intima (the lining of the artery), the potentially greater risk you have for heart disease.

❑ High-speed CT scan with calcium scoring: This is a CT scan assessing the amount of calcium in your heart vessels. The more calcium you have, the greater your risk for heart disease. You will need to speak with your physician about your test results.

You should discuss these recommendations with your physician to evaluate your need and the best type of test for you.

Optimal vital signs: You should regularly monitor these vital signs to ensure you are in the optimal range.

❑ Blood pressure: Optimal blood pressure is 120/70 or less. Take your blood pressure after resting for a few minutes. Keep your legs uncrossed and do not eat or drink two hours before testing since these can affect your blood pressure. Get an automated home blood pressure cuff to monitor your blood pressure at home if you feel that you may suffer from higher blood pressure at the doctor's office (referred to as "white coat hypertension").

❑ Weight: You want your BMI (body mass index) to be less than 25 (explained in Chapter Three).

❑ Body fat percentage: Optimally, I recommend that it be less than 10 percent for men and less than 20 percent for women.

❑ Waist circumference: The larger your waist, the greater your risk for heart disease. For men, an optimal waist is less than 35 inches. For women, an optimal waist is less than 30 inches.

OPTIMAL LAB VALUES
FROM YOUR BLOOD WORK

Laboratory assessments are an important part of your Optimal Health evaluation because they provide objective evidence of your baseline state of health as well as a trend of how you are doing over time. I provide trend sheets to all of my clients to help them track their improvements and areas where they need to continue to change.

It is important to realize that medicine is as much an art as it is a science. The "art" of Optimal Health is based on the common medical principle of risk modeling. In medicine, people with laboratory values that promote health (such as low cholesterol) are less likely to develop disease than people at higher levels of the same labs. In the state of Optimal Health, the reference ranges I use will always be ranges that are associated with lowering the probability of disease.

Optimal Health goals are evidence-based strategies to optimize your body, prevent health problems, and slow down aging. Thus, some of the laboratory tests I suggest are beyond the basic lab panels that traditional medicine offers.

Please remember that I am an Age Management Specialist. I evaluate laboratory tests differently from the traditional physician in order to help my patients achieve Optimal Health. Normal does not mean as much to me as Optimal does. Your primary care physician may not agree with obtaining some of the tests that I recommend below. Second, your physician may disagree with the optimal range because she or he is still evaluating labs within the traditional "normal" range. And third, traditional medicine believes aging is a normal process that leads to deficiencies, whereas I, as an Age Management Specialist, believe the deficiencies in many instances need to be safely replaced to improve health and slow the aging process that is occurring in all of us. I strongly believe that if we can optimize health, we will decrease the chronic disease that is afflicting our elderly population and reducing their quality of life.

LABS FOR OPTIMAL GLUCOSE CONTROL

Fasting Glucose

To diagnose diabetes with a fasting glucose level, you need a fasting glucose of 126 mg/dl or greater or a random blood glucose of 200 mg/dl.

Fasting Glucose			
Optimal Range	Normal Range	Borderline Diabetic Range	Diabetic
65-95 mg/dl	65-99 mg/dl	100-125 mg/dl	126 mg/dl

What are the risk factors for diabetes?
- 45 years old or above
- Overweight (BMI equal to or more than 25 kg/m2)
- Metabolic syndrome (see page 93)
- Family history of diabetes
- Habitual physical inactivity
- Race/ethnicity (African American, Hispanic, Native American, or South Asian)
- History of gestational diabetes or delivery of baby weighing 9 pounds or more
- Hypertension (equal to or greater than 135/85 mm Hg in adults)
- HDL (good cholesterol) less than 35 mg/dl and/or triglycerides equal to or greater than 250 mg/dl
- Polycystic ovarian syndrome (for women with some combination of irregular periods, acne, excess hair, and/or excess weight)
- History of cardiovascular disease

If you have at least two risk factors, you should have your hemoglobin A1c checked every six months to monitor your risk for developing diabetes. Keeping your hemoglobin A1c in the optimal range or close to it can prevent diabetes. Nutrition, exercise, and losing body fat as a "prescription" outperform every diabetic medication on the market today. I recommend the Mediterranean Diet (Chapter Three) and exercise (Chapter Four) regularly.

Hemoglobin A1c (HgA1c)

Hemoglobin A1c (HgA1c) or glycosylated hemoglobin is a test used to identify diabetes or your potential risk for developing diabetes as well as to assess your overall degree of dietary sugar consumption. For someone without diabetes, HgA1c will be less than 6 percent; anything above that should be considered a sign of diabetes. The fasting glucose test has been the standard for diagnosing and managing diabetes. While the fasting test remains an important part of diagnosis, its weakness is that it indicates your glucose level only at the moment you take the test. A fasting blood sugar doesn't tell you anything about your blood-sugar levels at other times. The hemoglobin A1c test provides your everyday average blood sugar over the past three to four months.

For Optimal Health, I recommend your HgA1c be less than 5 percent. This indicates that your dietary consumption of sugar is low, and your insulin levels will remain low. This allows you to lose more body fat as well as reduce the silent inflammation that causes us to age and develop chronic disease (more about this in Chapter Three).

Hemoglobin A1c				
Optimal Range	Normal Range	Average	Pre-diabetic	Diabetic
<5%	4-6%	5.1%-5.6%	5.7%-5.9%	6.0% and higher

Insulin

Insulin is the hormone that puts glucose into the cells where it is used for energy. As we will discuss in Chapter Three, high levels of insulin send a powerful signal to the brain to increase body fat. High insulin levels stimulate fat cells to make more fat and thus it becomes harder to lose weight. Keeping insulin as low as possible helps slow down the degenerative process that is occurring in all of us. For Optimal Heath, I recommend that insulin levels remain less than 5. High levels increase your risk for developing diabetes and heart disease. Insulin is not a standard test done by traditional physicians. Insulin levels must be done fasting for at least eight hours.

Insulin				
Optimal Range	Normal	Average	Pre-diabetic	Diabetic
1-5 ulU/ml	1-17 ulU/ml	6-12 ulU/ml	13-20 ulU/ml	>21 ulU/ml

LABS FOR ASSESSING CARDIOVASCULAR RISK

Cholesterol Panel

Your cholesterol profile is made of four different tests:

❑ Total Cholesterol: This is the combined total of the components below. You do need some cholesterol because it helps your body build cells and produce hormones necessary for life, but high levels increase your risk for heart disease. High cholesterol levels need to be assessed by the various components below.

Total Cholesterol		
Optimal Range	Normal Range	High Range
125-200 mg/dl	<200 mg/dl	>201 mg/dl

❑ HDL (high-density lipoprotein): HDL helps remove fat from your body by carrying it back to the liver for disposal. It is our "good" cholesterol which, if above 50 mg/dl, lowers our risk of heart disease and stroke. You can increase your HDL with exercise, losing weight, a Mediterranean Diet, and a daily glass of red wine. For many people, low HDL levels can be genetic, which increases heart disease risk. Women tend to have HDL higher levels, but after menopause, HDL levels fall and can increase the risk for heart disease.

HDL		
Optimal Range	Normal Range	Low Range
50-200 mg/dl	>40 mg/dl	<49 mg/dl

❑ LDL (low-density lipoprotein): The LDL cholesterol carries mostly fat and a small amount of protein from the liver to other parts of the body. Our "bad cholesterol," it increases our risk for heart disease. Optimal goals are less than 100 mg/dl; if you have heart disease, the goal is less than 70 mg/dl.

Some people, through diet and genetics, are able to keep their LDL cholesterol low, but many people will need to follow the Mediterranean Diet (Chapter Three), use supplements, and/or use a cholesterol-lowering medication if they are at high risk. Statins, the most effective prescribed cholesterol-reducing medication, can also decrease silent inflammation (see Chapter Three) and your risk of heart disease.

LDL		
Optimal Range	Medium Risk	High Risk
<100 mg/dl	101-130 mg/dl	>130 mg/dl
(<70 mg/dl if you have had heart disease)		

❏ Triglycerides: These are a type of fat the body uses to store energy. Having both high triglycerides and high LDL cholesterol increases your risk of heart disease more than just a high LDL cholesterol level. Bad fats (such as trans fats and saturated fats, explained in Chapter Three) tend to increase your triglyceride level. Some patients with genetic disorders have an increased triglyceride level. High triglyceride levels can be improved with a Mediterranean Diet, omega-3 fish oil or flaxseed, fiber, lots of fresh vegetables, and niacin. Optimal levels are less than 100 mg/dl, preferably less than 80 mg/dl.

Triglycerides		
Optimal Range	Normal Range	High Range
<100 mg/dl	<150 mg/dl	>101 mg/dl

Homocysteine

Homocysteine is an amino acid in your bloodstream. Excess accumulation leads to blood vessel damage, resulting in early stroke, atherosclerosis, and coronary heart disease. This risk factor is independent of your cholesterol levels. An estimated 10-20 percent of all cardiovascular disease is caused by excessive plasma homocysteine concentrations. It is estimated that 21 percent of the population is at increased or high risk.

Homocysteine	
Optimal Range	< 9.0 umoles/l
Normal Range	5.4-11.4 umoles/l

You are at risk for high homocysteine levels if you have or are
❖ a family history of atherosclerosis, heart disease (particularly at an early age), peripheral artery disease, stroke, high homocysteine levels
❖ a diet high in processed foods and low in fruits and vegetables
❖ a family history of Alzheimer's disease
❖ kidney disease or kidney failure
❖ high psychological stress
❖ hypothyroid
❖ diabetes
❖ rheumatoid arthritis
❖ an elderly or institutionalized adult
❖ a smoker
❖ postmenopausal.

The treatment is to take 800 mg to 1000 mg of folic acid daily, 100 mg of B6 daily, and 100 mg of B12 daily or as an injection once per month.

Cardio-CRP (C-Reactive Protein)

Cardio-CRP is a clinical indicator that measures silent inflammation around your heart (see page 52). High cardio-CRP levels indicate an increased risk for heart disease. Optimal levels should be below 1 mg/dl.

I recommend that your cardio-CRP levels be as low as possible. When you check these levels, please make sure you are not ill or have had any recent injuries since this can falsely elevate your cardio-CRP levels.

Cardio-CRP			
			Possible Inflammation
Optimal Range (Low Risk)	Medium Risk	High Risk	Elsewhere
0-1 mg/dl	1-3 mg/dl	3-10 mg/dl	>10 mg/dl

I recommend beginning with lifestyle changes if you are at medium risk and your LDL cholesterol (bad cholesterol) is less than 130. Follow a low glycemic diet, exercise regularly, and consume omega-3 fish oil. If you are at medium to high risk AND your LDL is greater than 130, speak with your physician about using a statin, a cholesterol-reducing medication, along with lifestyle changes as discussed above. CoQ10 and lycopene are two powerful antioxidants that can help decrease silent inflammation. I recommend repeating your test in two months to confirm it is decreasing.

LAB FOR ASSESSING YOUR RISK FOR OSTEOPOROSIS

Vitamin D Levels

Vitamin D levels are an important indicator of Optimal Health. Many recent medical journals have discussed the importance of Vitamin D not only for bone health, but for longevity, cardiovascular health, colon cancer prevention, and dental health. Optimal levels in the blood should be above 50 ng/ml with the best range being above 70 ng/ml. To achieve this, you need fifteen minutes of sun exposure and about 1000-2000 units of Vitamin D3 (also known as cholecalciferol). You should have your levels rechecked after a few months to ensure you are achieving optimal results. In Philadelphia, very few of my patients have optimal levels due to poor sun exposure.

Vitamin D			
Optimal Range	Deficient Levels	Low Levels	Normal Range
>50 ng/ml	<20 ng/ml	20-30 ng/ml	30 ng/ml and higher

OTHER IMPORTANT LABS

Ferritin

Ferritin levels measure your iron stores. Low levels of ferritin can be associated with fatigue, low energy, and hair loss. Low ferritin levels come from chronic bleeding within the digestive tract, heavy menstrual cycles, and after pregnancy. Levels above 70 ng/ml can help with energy and slow down hair loss if this is a concern for you. High ferritin levels can be due to liver disease, hemolytic anemias that cause destruction of the red blood cells, Hodgkins lymphoma (a blood cancer), acute inflammation from an illness or infection, or a disorder called hemochromoatosis in which your body tends to keep too much iron. Please speak with your doctor about possible causes of both high and low ferritin levels.

	Ferritin			
	Optimal Range	Too Low	Too High	Normal Range
Men	70-300 ng/ml	<70 ng/ml	>300 ng/ml	12-300 ng/ml
Women	70-150 ng/ml	<70 ng/ml	>150 ng/ml	15-150 ng/ml

Vitamin B12

Vitamin B12 is needed to produce healthy red blood cells, repair tissues and cells, synthesize DNA, and keep the neurological system functioning properly. Your body can store Vitamin B12 in your liver for three to five years, so a Vitamin B12 deficiency may take a few years to manifest.

A deficiency of Vitamin B12 can cause shortness of breath, fatigue, numbness and tingling, irritability, confusion, mouth sores, weakness, and hair loss as well as increase your risk for dementia and depression. Vitamin B12 is often low in patients with anemias, liver disease, alcoholism, digestive problems, or a strict vegetarian diet. Vitamin B12 can also decrease homocysteine levels (another independent risk factor for heart disease) and reduce the incidence of neural tube defects (spina bifida).

	Vitamin B12	
Optimal Range	Deficiency	Normal Range
700-900 pg/ml	<200 pg/ml	200-900 pg/ml

Vitamin B12 can be taken orally (100 mg daily) or by injection once per month. Vitamin B12 is found in meat products (three ounces of chicken), a glass of milk, or an egg.

Folic Acid

Folic acid is a B vitamin needed for cell replication and growth. Therefore, rapidly growing tissues, such as those of a fetus, and rapidly regenerating cells, like red blood cells and immune cells, have the highest need for folic acid.

Folic acid is found naturally in beans, leafy green vegetables, citrus fruits, beets, wheat germ, and meat. Low folic acid levels are associated with spina bifida, so it is important for women who are pregnant or trying to get pregnant. It is also a treatment for elevated homocysteine levels, alcoholism, liver disease, depression, abnormal pap smears, and may help with dementia, heart disease, stroke, and malabsorption disorders.

For Optimal Health, I recommend that your folic acid levels be greater than 20.

Folic Acid			
Optimal Range	Deficiency	Borderline	Normal Range
>20 ng/ml	<3.4 ng/ml	3.5-5.3 ng/ml	5.4-24 ng/ml

BUILDING SPOKE ONE
OF YOUR PERSONAL WELLNESS WHEEL™

Preventing chronic disease and maintaining Optimal Health is challenging. Most recommendations listed here need to be discussed with your physician to decide whether they apply to you. Developing a positive relationship with your physician is key for Optimal Health. I recommend forming a relationship with someone with whom you feel comfortable and who will review different options for treatment. You also need to listen to their concerns because they have your best interests in mind and know your personal health history. Achieving Optimal Health is an integration of your personal health habits and a pro-active, preventative approach to medicine. Following you will find trend sheets so you can track your progress.

OPTIMAL HEALTH LAB RESULTS

LAB NAME	Optimal Ranges	Date Done	Date Done	Date Done
HemoglobinA1c	4.0-5.0%			
Insulin	1-5 ulU/ml			
Fasting Glucose	65-95 mg/dl			
Total Cholesterol	<200 mg/dl			
Triglycerides	<100 mg/dl			
HDL	50-200 mg/dl			
LDL	70-100 mg/dl			
Cardio-CRP	0-1 mg/dl			
Homocysteine	1-9 umoles/l			
Vitamin D	50-70 ng/dl			
Vitamin B12	700-900 pg/ml			
Folic Acid	>20 ng/ml			
Ferritin	women: 70-150 ng/dl; men: 70-300 ng/dl			

OPTIMAL HEALTH RECORD FOR PREVENTATIVE MEDICINE

Test	Date Done	Date Done	Date Done
Pap Smear (women)			
Mammogram (women)			
Rectal Exam (yearly)			
Blood Stool Testing (yearly)			
Dexa Scan			
Eye Exam			
Dental Exam			
Skin Check (yearly)			
Colonoscopy			
Cardiac Stress Test			
Tetanus Vaccine			
Hepatitis B Vaccine			
Hepatitis A Vaccine			
Pneumoccal Vaccine			
Flu Vaccine			
Blood Pressure			
Weight Circumference (male <35"; women <30")			
Weight			
Height			
BMI (<25)			
Body Fat % (men 10% or less; women 20% or less)			

THE OPTIMAL HEALTH LIFESTYLE: CHANGING PERSONAL HABITS

A characteristic of human nature—perhaps the one that makes us most human—is our capacity to do the unnatural, to transcend and hence transform our own nature.

~ M. Scott Peck, MD

CONTENTS:
*smoking cessation
* alcohol, drugs, and any other addiction
* eating patterns
* getting enough sleep
* mental and emotional health
* building spoke two
* twenty question test on drug and alcohol problems
* optimal social habits record

The second spoke of your Personal Wellness Wheel™ gives you the information you need to make changes in your personal habits and to live the Optimal Heath lifestyle. A healthy lifestyle is one of the most important ways of slowing down the aging process. We build our Personal Wellness Wheels™ by the lives we live everyday. Good health has intrinsic momentum; when we feel good mentally, physically, and emotionally, we are more likely to engage in behaviors to improve health such as eating well, exercising, and living better. The spokes of the wheel work together, balancing one another to help us maintain the momentum of Optimal Health. However, many of us find it difficult to stop unhealthy habits, and therefore, we sabotage our goals—as much as we try, we just cannot get there.

For example, if you eat well, but cannot quit smoking, you are unable to put the whole wheel into practice. If you exercise, but continue to make poor food choices, you will sabotage your Optimal Health goals.

In this chapter, you will learn about the following:

○ Smoking Cessation

○ Alcohol, Drugs, and Any Other Addiction

○ Eating Patterns

○ Getting Enough Sleep

○ Mental and Emotional Health

SMOKING CESSATION

Smoking is one of worst things you can do for your health. You will not be able to create Optimal Health if you continue to smoke. Each time you pick up a cigarette, you risk your health and insure failure of your Personal Wellness Wheel™. Each cigarettes takes six minutes off your life. Whether you are a heavy, light, or social smoker, you need to stop. Secondhand smoke is unfortunately just as dangerous, so you need to convince your loved ones to quit smoking as well. If your exposure is work-related, you need to consider how you can separate yourself from it because it increases your risks of cancer, heart disease, respiratory infections, and chronic lung disease.

Here are some facts about the effects of smoking:

❖ Smoking affects almost every organ of the body. The Centers for Disease Control and Prevention (CDC) states that cigarette smoking accounts for an estimated 438,000 deaths, or nearly one of every five deaths, each year in the United States. More deaths are caused each year by tobacco use than by human immunodeficiency virus (HIV), illegal drug use, alcohol use, motor vehicle injury, suicide, and murder combined (CDC, 2002).

❖ Tobacco is one of the strongest cancer-causing agents known. Thirty percent of all cancer deaths in the United States are related to smoking. Smoking causes 90 percent of the lung cancers in men and women. Smoking increases the risk of cancers in the lung, throat, mouth, pancreas, kidney, bladder, and cervix. It is also associated with heart disease, strokes, peripheral vascular disease, emphysema, and bronchitis (CDC, 2004).

❖ Quitting smoking is not easy, but it can be done. Most health problems related to smoking can be reduced by stopping. Quitting smoking is beneficial at all ages, and the earlier you quit, the greater the benefits. Men who quit smoking by age 50 reduce their risk of lung cancer by almost two-thirds compared with men who continued to smoke to age 75 (CDC, 2002).

Fortunately, today there are many tools to help you quit. You can win the battle against smoking. What form you pick will be a personal preference, but all forms have been shown to be effective in 50-70 percent of the cases.

TOOLS TO QUIT SMOKING

Nicotine Patch

The nicotine patch provides a steady release of nicotine. It is a small, self-adhesive patch that slowly releases nicotine into the bloodstream through the outer layer of skin. It can be applied anywhere between the waist and neck—often on the upper arm or shoulder. Patches must be replaced every twenty-four hours. To minimize potential skin irritation, avoid putting the patch in the same place more than once every two weeks or so. Brand names: Nicoderm CQ® and Habitrol®. Generic patches are also available.

Nicotine Gum

Nicotine gum can control the oral urge to smoke by giving you something to chew. It can satisfy immediate cravings and comes in many flavors. Brand names include Nicorette® and Thrive™. Generic gum is also available.

Nicotine Lozenges

Nicotine lozenges can be used to quickly satisfy cravings. Nicotine lozenges are like eating hard candy. You place them between your gum and cheek and suck them slowly. Each lozenge lasts twenty to thirty minutes. Lozenges are sold under the brand name Commit®.

Nicotine Inhaler

The nicotine inhaler allows you to mimic the hand-to-mouth motions of smoking. The nicotine inhaler is a device that allows you to receive low doses of nicotine absorbed through the lining of your mouth and throat. Prescription: brand name Nicotrol®.

Nicotine Nasal Spray

The nicotine in nasal spray reaches the bloodstream more quickly than the other nicotine replacement medications. You spray the nicotine inside your nostrils. The recommended dose is a spray in each nostril from one up to five times per hour. Prescription: brand name Nicotrol®.

Varenicline

Varenicline is a medication that doesn't contain nicotine. Varenicline can help control cravings for tobacco and nicotine and withdrawal symptoms. It also blocks nicotine receptors in your brain, which in turn reduces the response to nicotine that you get from smoking a cigarette. Varenicline is available by prescription. Varenicline is sold in the United States under the brand name Chantix®.

Bupropion

Bupropion is a prescription stop-smoking aid that doesn't contain nicotine. Bupropion can decrease nicotine cravings. It's available under the brand name Zyban.

Hypnosis

Many people report that hypnosis helped them quit smoking. In these sessions, a practitioner will put you into a deep state of relaxation, which helps your unconscious mind to be open to suggestions. The practitioner then makes a series of suggestions on how to quit. Typically three to five sessions are required.

Cold Turkey

Many smokers have been able to quit "cold turkey." This means choosing a date, and on that date, stopping smoking. This is difficult for many people for obvious reasons.

No matter which way you choose to quit, do it today. The rewards are well worth it. You will then be able to fully engage in your Optimal Health lifestyle, free from smoking.

ALCOHOL, DRUGS, AND ANY OTHER ADDICTION

Today, rates of alcoholism and drug addiction are high in our country. To truly maintain a lifestyle of Optimal Health, you need to evaluate your alcohol, drug use, and other addictions. If you discover you have a problem, there are many ways to get treatment. The first is committing to an Optimal Health lifestyle, which means balance and moderation, especially in personal habits.

ALCOHOL

While there is nothing wrong with a glass of wine, drinking excessively will destroy your health. Drinking is part of our culture, yet it can be an unhealthy habit. A serving of alcohol is

- ❖ 12 ounces of regular beer or wine cooler
- ❖ 8 ounces of malt liquor
- ❖ 5 ounces of wine
- ❖ 1.5 ounces of 80-proof distilled spirits or liquor (e.g., gin, rum, vodka, whiskey).

If you do drink, limit your intake to one serving of alcohol. However, many people either binge drink or drink heavily. Binge drinking is:

- ❖ For women, four or more drinks during a single occasion.
- ❖ For men, five or more drinks during a single occasion.

Heavy drinking is

- ❖ For women, more than one drink per day on average.
- ❖ For men, more than two drinks per day on average.

The best drink you can have is red wine; beer is the worst. The glycemic index (which we will discuss in the next chapter) of beer is worse than that of sugar. It does not matter whether the beer is "light" or regular. If you are seriously interested in Optimal Health, neither beer or hard liquor is recommended. If you want a drink, have a small glass of red wine.

DRUGS

Many people use drugs recreationally. However, the Optimal Health lifestyle has no place for recreational drug use. This includes:

- ❖ Marijuana
- ❖ Cocaine
- ❖ Heroin

❖ Ecstasy

❖ Methamphetamine

❖ Any other mind-altering drug.

Many people today have also developed addictions to painkillers. Often, they have been prescribed for an injury or surgery, but the risk of dependency is high and may result in a dangerous addiction that needs professional treatment.

If you wonder whether you have a drinking or drug problem, ask yourself the following questions:

❖ Do you lose time from work due to drinking or drug use?

❖ Is drinking or drug use making your home life unhappy?

❖ Do you drink or use drugs because you are shy with other people?

❖ Is drinking or drug use affecting your reputation?

❖ Have you gotten into financial difficulties as a result of drinking or drug use?

❖ Have you ever felt remorse after drinking or drug use?

❖ Do you turn to different companions and environments when drinking or using drugs?

❖ Does your drinking or drug use make you careless of your family's welfare?

❖ Has your ambition decreased since drinking or using drugs?

❖ Do you crave a drink or drugs at a definite time daily?

❖ Do you want a drink or drugs the next morning?

❖ Does drinking or using drugs cause you to have difficulty sleeping?

❖ Has your efficiency decreased since drinking or using drugs?

❖ Is drinking or using drugs jeopardizing your job or business?

❖ Do you drink or use drugs to escape from worries or trouble?

❖ Do you drink or use drugs alone?

❖ Have you ever had a complete loss of memory as a result of drinking or drug use?

❖ Has your physician ever treated you for drinking or drug use?

❖ Do you drink or use drugs to build up your self-confidence?

❖ Have you ever been to a hospital or institution on account of drinking or drug use?

If you have answered yes to three or more questions, you may have a problem with alcohol or drugs. There are many ways to get help; ask your doctor about options.

SOME SUGGESTIONS FOR HELP
WITH ALCOHOL OR DRUG PROBLEMS

Alcoholics Anonymous

This peer program has consistently been most successful in helping people with alcoholism. People gather for "meetings," where they share their stories and support each other in recovery from their addictions. The program uses the twelve-step approach as a guide to living a sober life.

Narcotics Anonymous

This peer program has been effective in helping people deal with drug addiction. It is based on peer support, meetings, and a twelve-step approach.

Rehabilitation and Treatment

These are often twenty-eight day inpatient treatment programs known as "rehabs" where people learn about their addictions and are able to fully concentrate on recovery.

Drug Therapy

Drug treatments today can help people deal with some of the most difficult addictions, such as Oxycodone, heroin, painkillers, and alcohol. Subutex® and Suboxone® are among the treatments. You need to see a medical doctor who specializes in addiction treatments.

Psychotherapy

You may want to engage the services of a psychotherapist to talk about your alcohol and drug use. Consult your mental health coverage for a therapist or ask your friends who have seen a therapist for a personal referral.

Employee Assistance Programs (EAP)

Today, many of our workplaces offer programs to help people deal with addictions and mental health issues. Check with your Human Resources department to see what your employer offers.

Today there is no stigma to getting help for addictions, please be honest with yourself if you suspect you have a problem.

OTHER ADDICTIONS

There are other addictions besides alcohol and drugs. They are (but not limited to):

❖ Gambling

❖ Sex

❖ Food

❖ Shopping.

You can use the twenty question test on page 38 to determine whether you have a problem or to ask yourself if any of the behaviors above cause you to feel out of control or create problems in your life or your relationships.

EATING PATTERNS

Food can be an addiction too. Many times we eat because we "feel" like it or need comfort, not because we are genuinely hungry; this is called emotional eating. It adds unnecessary calories to our diets and makes it much more difficult to achieve Optimal Health—and stick to the goals presented in the third spoke of the Personal Wellness Wheel™ (Nutrition).

A good exercise to help you deal with emotional or comfort eating is to keep a food journal. Be honest! At the end of the day, record everything you have eaten that day. Next to each entry, write why you ate that particular food. After reviewing your choices at the end of each day, you will begin to see your eating patterns. You will find that many of the foods you ate were to provide comfort, were because you were bored, or were simply eaten out of habit.

> ### Try the following exercise when you are about to eat something:
> ❖ Recognize why you eat.
> ❖ Connect the "why" with what you are eating.
> ❖ Look at the food you are about to eat.
> ❖ Say aloud the reason why you are eating it, e.g., I am angry, lonely, bored, frustrated, anxious.
> ❖ Put the food down and walk away.
> ❖ Feel the feeling you are trying to stuff with food.
> ❖ Remember, the feeling is just a feeling. It won't harm you, but excessive eating will.

<u>**Also, do the following:**</u>

❖ Get rid of all unhealthy foods in your house, and do not buy them! You have a much better chance of following your diet plan if these foods are not in your home and you commit to not buying them!

❖ Change your nighttime habits. If you know you like to eat at night, try a new plan. Plan your exercise routine at night, read a book, or plan a creative project instead. Choose something that will distract you from food until the habit is broken.

❖ If you like to snack at work, choose something from the diet plan (see Chapter Three) and eat that. Do not bring candy, chips, or any calorie-laden foods to work!

❖ If you find that you cannot break your food habits or are eating to calm your emotions, you may want to talk to a therapist. You may need to look at and work through emotional issues. Once you do, you will find many of the "reasons" you ate are no longer there.

❖ When you feel a craving, drink a glass of water first. Sometimes what we perceive as hunger is actually thirst.

GETTING ENOUGH SLEEP

Sleep is a very important aspect of Optimal Health. In our society today, we almost pride ourselves on getting by with the fewest hours of sleep. But sleep is the only time when your body truly rests and regenerates itself.

We know from the medical literature that people who have difficulty sleeping report poor performance at work, memory difficulties, concentration problems, and twice as many fatigue-related automobile accidents as good sleepers. Poor sleep affects emotional and mental well-being as well. Poor sleep increases negative moods and irritability and can worsen mental health disorders.

Lack of sleep has also been shown to worsen chronic medical conditions. In 2003 a large study published in the *Archives of Internal Medicine* showed that women who slept less than five hours a night were 45 percent more likely to have heart problems than women who slept eight hours. The exact cause of increased heart attacks and strokes is not known, but it is hypothesized that an increase in stress hormones triggers the adverse event.

Sleep deprivation can affect how your body processes blood sugar, which can raise your risk of diabetes. One 1999 *Lancet* study of eleven healthy, young men found that after just six days of sleeping for four hours a night, their insulin and blood sugar levels were similar to those of people on the verge of diabetes. Furthermore, a recent report by the American Academy of Sleep Medicine stated that poor sleep has been linked with poor diets. People who sleep poorly are more likely to eat out and choose foods that are unhealthy, resulting in weight gain, which increases the risk for diabetes and heart disease.

Researchers have also found that sleep deprivation can interfere with the ability to lose weight. There appears to be a physiological reason. Leptin is a hormone produced by fat cells and is an appetite suppressant; grehlin is produced by the stomach and is an appetite stimulant. Grehlin and leptin are opposites in their effect on appetite. When grehlin is high, leptin is low. Research has shown that with sleep deprivation, grehlin levels are elevated and leptin levels are depressed, resulting in an increased appetite without ever feeling full. This may help explain some of the weight gain seen in shift workers, stressed individuals, and the college student's "freshmen fifteen."

Common Types of Sleep Disorders

Insomnia

Insomnia is a significant lack of high-quality sleep; it can be either a short-term or a chronic problem. Insomnia can be caused by stress, a change in time zones or sleep schedule, poor bedtime habits, or an underlying medical or psychiatric condition.

In most cases, insomnia can be helped by improving bedtime habits, relieving stress, and relaxation exercises. However, certain medications may be prescribed by your doctor if these alternative treatments do not have the desired effect.

Sleep Apnea

Sleep apnea is a common disorder that can be very serious and even life-threatening. When you have sleep apnea, your breathing stops or gets very shallow while you are sleeping. Each pause in breathing typically lasts ten to twenty seconds or more. These pauses can occur twenty to thirty times or more an hour. Symptoms include frequent waking episodes at night, usually accompanied by a feeling of "choking" or gasping for air. Your significant other will report hearing gasping, gagging, or choking sounds. Treatment may include behavioral changes, physical and mechanical devices, and in some cases, surgery.

Restless Legs Syndrome (RLS)

Restless legs syndrome (RLS) is a sensory disorder causing an almost irresistible urge to move the legs due to uncomfortable, tingly, or creeping sensations that occur when at rest.

Narcolepsy

Narcolepsy is a disorder that results in difficulty in staying awake. Narcolepsy may cause a person to suddenly fall asleep during the day, even after getting enough sleep. Falling asleep during activities like walking, driving, cooking, or talking can have dangerous consequences with regard to safety as well as professional and personal performance.

If you feel you have a sleeping disorder, discuss with your physician the evaluation and management of this problem. Follow these simple ideas to help you maintain better sleep:

TIPS FOR GOOD SLEEP

❖ **Good sleep is an important aspect of Optimal Health.** Both the quality and quantity of sleep are important. Most adults need between 7.5 to 8.5 hours of uninterrupted sleep.

❖ **Keep regular hours.** Try to go to bed and get up at the same time every day. Getting up at the same time is most important. Getting bright light, like the sun, when you get up will also help. Try to go to bed only when you are sleepy.

❖ **Avoid caffeine, nicotine, and alcohol**. This will help you get deep sleep, which is the most refreshing. If you take any caffeine, do so in the morning. Avoid all stimulants in the evening, including chocolate, caffeinated sodas, caffeinated teas, nicotine, or alcohol. They will delay sleep and increase arousal during the night.

❖ **Use the bed for sleeping (and sex) only.** Avoid watching TV or using laptop computers. Know that reading in bed can be a problem if the material is very stimulating and you read with a bright light. If it helps to read before sleep, make sure you use a very small wattage bulb; a fifteen watt bulb should be enough. Bright light from these activities may inhibit sleep.

❖ **Avoid bright light around the house before bed.** Using dimmer switches in living rooms and bathrooms before bed can be helpful.

❖ **Manage your stress because it affects your sleep.** Participate in yoga or tai chi; try our meditation CD. Read Chapter Seven for more information.

❖ **Get regular exercise, but not near bedtime.** Do not exercise at least three hours before bed. Regular exercise at other times, though, helps create physical fatigue which can help with deep sleep.

❖ **Bedtime routines are helpful for good sleep.** Keep routines on your normal schedule. A cup of herbal tea an hour before bed or meditation before you sleep can help clear your mind.

❖ **If you can't get to sleep for over thirty minutes, get out of bed and do something boring in dim light until you are sleepy.**

❖ **Keep your bedroom at a comfortable temperature,** not too warm and not too cold. Cooler is better than warmer.

❖ **Stop excess noise by your bedroom.** If loud noises disturb your sleep, try ear plugs or a fan to help block the noise. Those who are sensitive to magnetic forces can try moving all electrical equipment that is close to the bed to the other side of the room.

❖ **If you have a sleeping partner, ask if she or he notices any snoring, leg movements, and/or pauses in your breathing.** You may have a sleep disorder about which you need to see your doctor.

MENTAL AND EMOTIONAL HEALTH

Good mental health is an important component of your Personal Wellness Wheel™. Eastern philosophy believes that the body, mind, and spirit are connected. This means that your mind and your response to the events around you play a role in your Optimal Health. They are not separate from your body.

In the seventh spoke, we will address, in depth, how meditation can calm your mind and how to use our techniques for stress management.

But in this spoke, we are concerned with mental health with regard to depression and anxiety. Depression affects many people today, and many treatments are available. Often, mild symptoms of depression are eliminated when you put your Personal Wellness Wheel™ into action. Changing your diet, exercising, optimizing your hormones, and optimizing your lab values may lead to better mental and emotional health.

However, if you experience the following symptoms persistently, you should talk to your doctor about available treatments.

❖ Depressed or irritable mood most of the day, nearly every day

❖ Loss of interest or pleasure in activities (such as hobbies, work, sex, or being with friends) most of the day, nearly every day

❖ A sudden change in weight (weight loss without dieting or gaining more than 5 percent of body weight in one month) or a change in appetite

❖ Inability to sleep or sleeping too much, nearly every day

❖ Agitation or restlessness (observed by others), nearly every day

❖ Constant fatigue or loss of energy, nearly every day

❖ Frequent feelings of worthlessness or inappropriate guilt, nearly every day

❖ Difficulty concentrating or making decisions, nearly every day

Anxiety affects millions of people and is sometimes called GAD or Generalized Anxiety Disorder. This needs to be properly diagnosed, but if you suffer from three or more of the following symptoms and they are present for over half the days in the past six months, you may have GAD.

❖ Feeling restless, edgy, keyed up
❖ Tiring easily
❖ Trouble concentrating
❖ Irritability
❖ Increased muscle tension
❖ Trouble sleeping (initial insomnia or restless, unsatisfying sleep)
❖ Excessive anxiety and worry about several events or activities for more than half the days for at least six months
❖ Trouble controlling these feelings

Many of these symptoms may be eliminated through following the spokes on your Personal Wellness Wheel™ and following your Optimal Health Program. If they persist, however, you should consult your doctor about treatment options.

There are many good anti-depressants today with minor side effects which, in combination with psychotherapy, may help if you have a serious depression or anxiety.

BUILDING SPOKE TWO
OF YOUR PERSONAL WELLNESS WHEEL™

Lifestyle changes are extremely important in maintaining your Personal Wellness Wheel™. You can make changes in your diet, exercise, and have good lab values, but if you continue to smoke or drink excessively, you will not achieve Optimal Health. But with this holistic approach to health and well-being, I believe each person can change, improve, and become a better, stronger person. More importantly, you are worth changing for!

Here are some tips for building this spoke of your Personal Wellness Wheel™.

❑ If you smoke, resolve to quit. Write down your plan for quitting:

_____

_____

_____

❑ Use the Twenty Question Test on page 48 to determine whether you have a drug or alcohol issue.

 ❑ Evaluate other possible addictions (gambling, food, sex, shopping) by using the Twenty Question Test.

❑ Eating Patterns:

 ❖ Use a food journal to help you to determine your eating patterns.

 ❖ Use the following exercise when you are about to eat something:

 ◆ Connect the why with what you are eating.

 ◆ Look at the food you are about to eat.

 ◆ Say aloud the reason why you are eating it, e.g., I am angry, lonely, frustrated, anxious.

 ◆ Put the food down and walk away.

 ◆ Feel the feeling you are trying to stuff with food.

 ◆ Remember, the feeling is just a feeling. It won't harm you, but excessive eating will.

❑ Sleeping Patterns:
- ❖ Sleep seven to eight hours each night.
- ❖ Go to bed and get up at the same time every day.
- ❖ Avoid caffeine, nicotine, and alcohol in the afternoon and evening.
- ❖ Use your bed for sleeping (and sex) only.
- ❖ Avoid bright light around the house before bed.
- ❖ Manage your stress.
- ❖ Get regular exercise but not near bedtime.
- ❖ Keep your bedroom at a comfortable temperature.
- ❖ Stop excess noise by or in your bedroom.

❑ Depression/Anxiety

As a baseline for your Personal Wellness Wheel™, check if you have the following symptoms.
- ❖ Depressed or irritable mood most of the day, nearly every day
- ❖ Loss of interest or pleasure in activities (such as hobbies, work, sex, or being with friends) most of the day, nearly every day
- ❖ A sudden change in weight (weight loss without dieting or gaining more than 5 percent of body weight in one month) or a change in appetite
- ❖ Inability to sleep or sleeping too much, nearly every day
- ❖ Agitation, irritability, or restlessness (observed by others), nearly every day
- ❖ Constant fatigue or loss of energy, nearly every day
- ❖ Frequent feelings of worthlessness or inappropriate guilt, nearly every day
- ❖ Difficulty concentrating or making decisions, nearly every day
- ❖ Feeling edgy, keyed up
- ❖ Trouble concentrating
- ❖ Increased muscle tension
- ❖ Excessive anxiety and worry about several events or activities for more than half the days in at least six months
- ❖ Trouble controlling these feelings

Many of these symptoms may resolve after you practice your Personal Wellness Wheel™.

TWENTY QUESTION TEST ON DRUG OR ALCOHOL PROBLEMS

❖ Do you lose time from work due to drinking or drug use?

❖ Is drinking or drug use making your home life unhappy?

❖ Do you drink or use drugs because you are shy with other people?

❖ Is drinking or drug use affecting your reputation?

❖ Have you gotten into financial difficulties as a result of drinking or drug use?

❖ Have you ever felt remorse after drinking or drug use?

❖ Do you turn to different companions and environments when drinking or using drugs?

❖ Does your drinking or drug use make you careless of your family's welfare?

❖ Has your ambition decreased since drinking or using drugs?

❖ Do you crave a drink or drugs at a definite time daily?

❖ Do you want a drink or drugs the next morning?

❖ Does drinking or using drugs cause you to have difficulty sleeping?

❖ Has your efficiency decreased since drinking or using drugs?

❖ Is drinking or using drugs jeopardizing your job or business?

❖ Do you drink or use drugs to escape from worries or trouble?

❖ Do you drink or use drugs alone?

❖ Have you ever had a complete loss of memory as a result of drinking or drug use?

❖ Has your physician ever treated you for drinking or drug use?

❖ Do you drink or use drugs to build up your self-confidence?

❖ Have you ever been to a hospital or institution because of drinking or drug use?

If you have answered yes to three or more questions, you may have a problem with alcohol or drugs. There are many ways to get help; ask your doctor about options.

This test can also be used to determine if you may have a problem with another addiction, such as gambling; just substitute that issue for "drinking or drug use" in the above questions.

OPTIMAL SOCIAL HABITS RECORD

Name:

Habits	Dates: How <u>much</u> per day or week? How <u>often</u> per day or week?	Dates: How <u>much</u> per day or week? How <u>often</u> per day or week?	Dates: How <u>much</u> per day or week? How <u>often</u> per day or week?
Smoking Cigarettes *Optimally 0*			
Smoking Cigars *Optimally 0*			
Smoking Other *Optimally 0*			
ALCOHOL <u>Wine</u> *Optimally 1 glass per day (or less)* <u>Beer</u> *Optimally 0* <u>Hard Liquor</u> *Optimally 0*			
DRUGS <u>Types:</u> *Optimally 0*			

YOUR FUEL FOR LIFE: CREATING ULTIMATE NUTRITION

Let food be your medicine and medicine be your food.

~ Hippocrates

Nutrition

provides the energy you need for everything from small, daily tasks like blinking to major efforts like running marathons. Your body uses the nutrition you give it as the fuel or energy needed at the cellular level to remain healthy, fight off illness, and slow degeneration. In addition, nutrition accounts for almost 50 percent of the cause of all chronic disease and thus is a powerful spoke of change. Nutrition affects us on a daily basis and can be one of the most effective and long-lasting ways of reaching Optimal Health and slowing the aging process.

In this chapter, you will learn about the following:

- Types of Inflammation
- Proteins
- Fats
- Carbohydrates and Sugars
- Other
- Supplements
- Fluids
- Eating Well is a Lifestyle
- The Mediterranean Diet

TYPES OF INFLAMMATION

Degeneration of our bodies results from inflammation. There are two types of inflammation. The first (which occurs at all ages) is your body's general response when hurt or exposed to an illness, toxins, or allergies. Your body sends a powerful message to the brain to heal itself; inflammation results so your body can protect and heal itself.

The second type of inflammation, a chronic, low-grade inflammation that goes undetected by the body, is called **silent inflammation**. Scientists believe that this low-grade inflammation causes us to degenerate constantly. Silent inflammation causes many of the chronic diseases associated with aging: osteoporosis, Alzheimer's disease, hypertension, type 2 diabetes, cancer, stroke, heart disease, insulin resistance, and a suppressed immune system. It also accelerates the aging process (including changes such as wrinkles and age spots) and causes loss of muscle mass. The body does not see this inflammation as needing repair, and thus these degenerative changes occur slowly.

Building this spoke in your Personal Wellness Wheel™ will help you fight this silent inflammation and give you an easy way to get the best possible nutrition for Optimal

GUIDELINES FOR CHOOSING PROTEIN

- **Consume healthy proteins:**
  - o White meat: chicken and turkey (without the skin)
  - o Salmon, tuna, trout, and other cold-water fish (recommended at least three to four times a week)
  - o Whole eggs (two to four per week, preferably omega-3 enriched) and egg whites
  - o Soybeans (also called edamame)
  - o Tofu
  - o Low-fat dairy products (such as cottage cheese and yogurt)
- **Ingest more proteins from plant sources.** The more plant-based our diet becomes, the healthier it is.
- **Eat organic or grass-fed meats.**
- **Increase the soy protein** you eat to 25 grams per day. Together with a low-fat diet, this can reduce cardiovascular disease by reducing inflammation.
- **Limit your intake of**
  - o dark meat chicken and turkey, lean cuts of beef, ham, pork, and lean Canadian bacon. You should eat red meat and pork at most one to two times per month.
  - o fatty cuts of meat (including hot dogs, bacon, sausage, and liver, as well as hard cheeses).

Health.

The first step in building this spoke is to educate yourself about the elements of what constitutes good nutrition so that you can begin to make good choices every day.

PROTEINS

Proteins are essential for your body's structure and proper function. They function as enzymes (to speed up processes such as digestion), hormones, and antibodies (made when your body responds to an exposure such as hepatitis or vaccines) and are used for transport and structural components.

FATS

Dietary fat is a main cause of silent inflammation, specifically a diet low in monounsaturated fats and omega-3s, but high in trans fats, saturated fats, and polyunsaturated fats.

So what does this mean? There are two types of fat: saturated and unsaturated. Unsaturated fats are further divided into three subcategories: trans fats, monounsaturated fats (including omega-9s), and polyunsaturated fats (composed of omega-3 and omega-6 fats, also called the essential fatty acids [EFA] because our bodies cannot manufacture them and so we need to get them through our diet). Basically, saturated fats are bad fats; for Optimal Health, it is best to avoid them as much as possible.

BAD FATS

Saturated Fats

Saturated fats are bad for you because they increase your total and "bad" cholesterol (LDL). Your total cholesterol is made of bad cholesterol (LDL), good cholesterol (HDL), and triglycercides (another type of measurement that is affected by bad dietary fats and/or our bodies converting excess bad carbohydrates to fat).

Saturated fats should make up only 10 percent of our diet or none at all. If you do eat red meat, try to eat grass-fed or organic meats. Grass-fed meats are from animals that were fed their mother's milk or only grass and hay. Be careful with the label "free-range." There is no current government regulation as to how long the animals are allowed to range freely; it can be one hour to all day. The best way to know is to contact your meat distributor for information.

Trans Fats

Trans fats are vegetable oils that have undergone a process called hydrogenation. This enables them to remain solid at room temperature and allows foods cooked with them to have a longer shelf-life. They are artificial and the worst fat for us. How good can something be if it can be stored indefinitely—like a bag of cookies?

Why are they so bad? Trans fats exponentially increase your risk for heart disease because while they increase your total and "bad" (LDL) cholesterol, they decrease your natural protection against heart disease: your "good" cholesterol (HDL). They also increase silent inflammation which again accelerates your degenerative process. Furthermore, they stop you from absorbing good fats (such as omega-3s) that can help slow down the aging process!

The American diet is composed of about 4 to 7 percent trans fats. Our diets should be ZERO percent trans fat. Trans fats are found in processed foods, baked goods, store-bought cookies, cakes, crackers, chips, margarine, and restaurant frying oils.

GOOD FATS

Monounsaturated Fats

There *are* good sources of fats—and your body needs them to work optimally. These fats are essential for slowing aging and enabling all the systems of your body to work together.

Monounsaturated fats are good fats. Monounsaturated fats actually decrease your risk of heart disease because they are anti-inflammatory and have very strong antioxidant properties.

Monounsaturated fats are also called omega-9s. They come in olive oil (extra virgin is best) and canola oil. Olive oil is a great source of natural Vitamin E and polyphenols (substances that act like antioxidants) that reduce inflammation in the cardiovascular system. Canola oil is also an excellent monounsaturated oil.

Besides these oils, nuts are a wonderful source of monounsaturated oils. Omega-9s are found in pistachios, cashews, almonds, pecans, and macadamias. Avocados are also very high in monounsaturated fats, so enjoy them.

Polyunsaturated Fats

The next category of good fats is polyunsaturated fats, composed of omega-3 and omega-6 fats. But there is a difference.

Omega-3 fats are excellent. They have antioxidant, anti-thrombotic, and anti-inflammatory properties. Omega-3s help reduce inflammation, prevent life-threatening heart rhythm irregularities, cancers of the prostate, breast, and colon, Crohn's disease, and Alzheimer's disease; inhibit atherosclerosis (the build-up of plaque on artery walls); improve depression and Attention Deficit Hyperactivity Disorder (ADHD); help with neonatal brain development; reduce blood pressure, cholesterol, and triglycerides; and improve blood vessel health and skin appearance (including reducing acne).

Omega-3s come in three types: Eicosapentaenoic acid (EPA), Docosahexaenoic acid (DHA), and Alpha-linolenic acid (ALA). EPA and DHA are marine sources (from cold-water fish such as salmon, tuna, trout, sardines, and mackerel or algae [for DHA]); ALA are plant sources (from soybeans, tofu, flax seed, walnuts, and leafy green vegetables). EPA and DHA found in marine sources are much more effective in reducing inflammation.

Omega-6 fats are found in vegetable oils, corn oil, safflower oil, sunflower oil, cottonseed oil, seeds, baked goods, poultry, and cheese. Too much omega-6 fat can cause blood clots and inflammation. Americans consume large amounts of vegetable oils that are very high in omega-6 fatty acids. Additionally, domesticated animals in this country are fed very large amounts of omega-6 fatty acids, so when we consume meat, we ingest additional omega-6.

The ratio of omega-6 fatty acids to omega-3 fatty acids in the American diet is 20 to 1. In the early human diet, it was 1 or 2 to 1. A ratio of 10 or more to 1 puts us at high risk for inflammation and thrombosis—the cause of most heart attacks and strokes

So how much do we need? For heart protection, we need one gram per day of EPA and DHA (added together). We need two to four grams per day to reduce elevated triglycerides and morning stiffness.

CARBOHYDRATES AND SUGARS

SUGARS

Most of us know that overt sugars are bad; doctors and nutritionists—and maybe our moms—have told us to eliminate or cut back on sodas, candy bars, and more. But that is not the only place sugars hide. Most people are surprised to learn about the more "hidden" forms of sugars in many of our favorite and staple foods. These sugars have a lot to do with degeneration—and thus contribute to keeping us from Optimal Health. This is especially important because a lot of marketing tries to sell us "healthy" foods that are actually loaded with sugar. Be sure to look at food labels to check for hidden sugars, and avoid these foods.

CARBOHYDRATES

Carbohydrates provide energy in the form of glucose. The good carbohydrates have fiber and are complex, such as vegetables, fruits, and whole grains. These improve our cholesterol and maintain our weight. The "bad carbohydrates" are foods easily broken down and immediately converted to glucose. They are usually processed and refined foods that have overt and hidden sugars in them. They can cause weight gain, increase cholesterol, and form disease. We want to avoid these. So stop thinking about all carbs as being bad, but do understand that there are good carbs and bad carbs.

THE GLYCEMIC INDEX

The glycemic index (GI) ranks carbohydrates (gram for gram) based on their immediate effect on blood glucose (blood sugar) levels. Carbohydrates that break down quickly during digestion have high glycemic indices—your blood glucose goes screaming up as soon as you eat.

Carbohydrates that break down slowly, thus releasing glucose gradually into the bloodstream, have low glycemic indices. With a low GI diet, your glucose and insulin levels remain low. You can efficiently burn fat and lose weight. A low GI diet can improve your health. Foods that are low in the glycemic index do not cause the up-and-down fluctuation of glucose levels and insulin levels. If you follow a low glycemic index diet, your body can very efficiently burn fat, have more energy, and stay healthy.

A low GI diet can
❖ result in a smaller rise in blood glucose levels after meals
❖ help you lose weight
❖ improve your body's sensitivity to insulin
❖ improve diabetes control
❖ improve cholesterol
❖ keep you fuller longer and eliminate cravings
❖ help you with prolonged physical endurance.

THE GLYCEMIC LOAD

The glycemic load measures how much sugar you eat in a serving. For example, many of my health-conscious clients tell me, "I don't eat carrots or beets. They are just little sugar cubes because their glycemic index is high." However, their glycemic load is low. At the most, we usually only eat a handful of carrots or a beet. The total amount of sugar we eat is the glycemic load. The glycemic index is based on fifty grams of any food item. This is usually okay for common foods, but most people do not eat fifty grams of beets in a single sitting.

Now the question becomes: how do you know what a food's glycemic index or glycemic load is? One of the best Websites is www.glycemicindex.com. But generally, a good rule of thumb is that if it is found in nature, it probably has a low glycemic index, and typically the amount you want to eat is a palm size. The exceptions to this "Mother Nature rule" are potatoes, corn, tropical fruits (such as pineapple, mango, and papaya), melons (such as watermelon, honeydew, and cantaloupe), raisins, and all dried fruits except for apricots.

Low Glycemic Foods: Great Foods to Eat

Food Items	Serving size	Carbohydrate Content on label	Glycemic Index	Glycemic Load
Peanuts	50grams/2oz	6	14	1
Soy beans	150g/1 cup	6	18	1
Barley	150g/1 cup	42	25	11
Whole Milk	250g/1 cup	12	27	3
Kidney Beans	150g/1 cup	30	28	8
Chick Peas	150g/1 cup	25	28	7
All Bran Cereal	30g/0.5 cup	23	38	9
Lentils	150g/1 cup	18	29	5
Boiled Egg	1 egg	46	20	5

Medium Glycemic Foods:
Foods to Avoid Because of Their High GI and GL Content

Food Items	Serving size	Carbohydrate Content on label	Glycemic Index	Glycemic Load
Macaroni	180g/1.25cup	48	47	23
Orange Juice	250g/1 cup	26	50	13
Apple Juice	250g/1 cup	29	52	12
Linguine	180g/1.3cup	45	52	23
Banana	120g/each	24	52	12
Wild Rice	150g/1 cup	37	54	20
Pound Cake	53g/1 piece	28	54	15
Power Bar	65g/1 bar	42	56	54

High Glycemic Foods:
Avoid Completely Because They are Loaded with Sugar

Food Items	Serving Size	Carbohydrate Content on label	Glycemic Index	Glycemic Load
Popcorn	20g/2 cups	11	72	8
Jelly Beans	30g/1 oz	28	78	22
Wonder Bread	30g/1 slice	14	73	10
Baked Potato	1 potato	30	85	26
Corn Flakes	30g/1 cup	36	92	24

So What Foods Should I Eat?

We want to eat foods that have a glycemic index less than 55. If you are trying to lose weight, you want to eat foods that have a glycemic index less than 45.

	Glycemic Index	Glycemic Load
Low Range	<55	<10
Medium Range	56-69	11-19
High Range	>70	>20

Please note that all grains made from white flour or white rice are very high in the glycemic index. Thus, you want to eat only whole grains.

SUGAR ALTERNATIVES

If you do crave sugar, what can you do? The following are healthier substitutes for table sugar and artificial sweeteners.

- ❖ Agave nectar comes from the agave fruit, found mostly in Latin America. It has a lower glycemic index than sugar, and a small amount goes a very long way!
- ❖ Stevia comes from a Paraguayan plant and is 100 times sweeter than table sugar so use only a small amount!
- ❖ Real maple syrup comes from the concentrated sap of maple trees and is great for baking.
- ❖ Brown rice syrup is a slowly digested sugar alternative and is great for baking.
- ❖ Honey comes in many different types and textures. The more raw the honey, the better it is for you. Honey can also help with immunity and wound healing.

OTHER

FIBER

Research has shown that when we eat more than thirty grams of fiber per day, we decrease our risk of colorectal cancer, diabetes, and coronary artery disease. Dietary fiber reduces inflammation by slowing digestion and stomach emptying, which reduces the blood glucose and triglyceride spikes after eating. This reduces the formation of free radicals (byproducts formed from normal metabolism in our bodies that cause us to degenerate) which can reduce silent inflammation.

An easy way to get your fiber is to remember that a serving size is your hand in a cupped form. One serving of fruit, nuts, seeds, or veggies usually has about three grams of fiber. One piece of multigrain bread, oatmeal, or brown rice has about three to five grams of fiber as well. Some of the best cereals are Kellogg's® All-Bran® Original and Fiber One® Original, which both have fourteen grams of fiber per serving. Kashi is another great brand that has a low glycemic index and is rich in fiber.

Whole grains are a great source of fiber. Thinking that grain is just wheat will lead you to miss out on a lot! Expand your horizons and try different grains such as millet, quinoa, barley, oats, bran, or kamut.

GREEN FOODS

"Super green" foods are packed with antioxidants, minerals, and vitamins, along with chlorophyll, which is similar to hemoglobin's molecular structure and helps increase your circulation and energy. These green foods include wheat germ, barley, wheat grass, alfalfa, chlorella, spirulina, blue-green algae (AFA), and green tea.

PROTEIN BARS/SHAKES

Protein bars and shakes are commonly used to maintain and achieve good health. Protein shakes and bars are healthier when they combine whey and soy protein. You can call the manufacturing company to obtain the glycemic index of their product. But generally if a protein shake or powder has a total sugar level below ten, it is probably alright. To make it healthier, use water, milk, or (if you need juice) a small amount of apple juice or pomegranate juice with lots of fresh or frozen fruit.

SPICES

In Aruyveda, spices were used to prevent many diseases long before we had medications. Modern science has just begun to understand and appreciate the health benefits of spices.

Cayenne/chili has been used for centuries as a medicine. It can reduce the risk of cardiovascular disease by reducing cholesterol and triglyceride levels and blood clot formation. It has been used for digestive ailments like gas build-up and to relieve cramped muscles. Cayenne can be a powerful analgesic (pain reducer) and anti-inflammatory.

Cinnamon helps decrease the glucose spike after you eat by slowing down digestion. Cinnamon can stop the growth of unwanted bacteria, fungi, and yeast. It is a powerful antioxidant and has anti-clotting and anti-inflammatory properties, which help prevent unwanted blood platelet clumping. Cinnamon may also boost brain function.

Garlic, when regularly consumed, can decrease blood pressure and cholesterol levels. It aids digestion, prevents flatulence, and has antiseptic properties. Recent research shows garlic to be beneficial in treating diabetes. Garlic is an antioxidant and can combat free radicals in your body.

Ginger is good for the stomach. Drink ginger ale or chew on raw ginger to help with nausea or to calm an upset stomach. Ginger is also believed to reduce inflammation of the heart.

Oregano has two compounds—thymol and carvacrol—that have potent antibacterial properties. Oregano is a powerful antioxidant. On a per-gram basis, fresh oregano has forty-two times more antioxidant activity than apples, twelve times more than oranges, and four times more than blueberries.

Sesame seeds are a great source of calcium; one tablespoon has over 1000 mg of calcium—equivalent to three glasses of milk!

Parsley's beneficial properties include its ability to fight cancer. Parsley is also a rich source of antioxidants and heart-protective nutrients including Vitamin C, beta-carotene, and folic acid.

Turmeric is anti-inflammatory and helps fight inflammatory bowel diseases (including Crohn's disease and ulcerative colitis), rheumatoid arthritis, cystic fibrosis, cancer, and Alzheimer's disease. In India, Alzheimer's is relatively rare; it is believed that the turmeric used in Indian cooking is one of the reasons.

Vinegar decreases the after-eating glucose spike and increases the sensation of fullness.

SUPPLEMENTS

Supplements are another area that causes uncertainty among the general population and with physicians. As physicians, we receive very little formal education on nutrition or supplements. Furthermore, much of the information we do receive assumes that all people benefit from the same supplement or dose; that is just not true. The rationale for selective supplementation is that as we age, we begin to require replacement of important depleted factors.

Below is a list of common supplements to help maintain good health for men and women. Supplement needs can change if you have ongoing chronic medical conditions, but this is a general list. For more specific information, you should see your physician or visit us online for your individual consultation.

FOR WOMEN

Folic acid is an important supplement for women to begin three to four months prior to becoming pregnant to decrease the risk of spina bifida. Use about 400-800 mcg/day. After menopause it is important in the prevention of heart disease and may improve Alzheimer's.

CoQ10 is important for your body's ability to produce energy at any age. Use 100 mg daily. If you are training for an endurance sport such as a marathon or have a chronic disease, use 300 mg/day because your body needs to produce more energy for your extra workouts and/or disease process.

L Carnitine works with CoQ10 to help the energy cycle work faster. It helps bring long-chain fatty acids into the cell for energy and helps remove toxins and waste from your cells. It can also help with exercise tolerance, improve heart function and energy, and decrease cholesterol. I recommend it for healthy women over age 40 or earlier for those with a chronic disease.

Multivitamins must have about 5000 units of Vitamin A (to help with vision and skin renewal), calcium (1000 mg), magnesium (500 mg), trace amounts of selenium (for bone health), Vitamin E and C (good antioxidants, but you don't need to overdo them), and Vitamin B complex (for nerve health, mental health, and skin and hair health; especially important for vegetarians). I favor using a multivitamin because our hectic lives often prevent obtaining these in our daily lives. A good multivitamin can help.

Omega-3 fish oil is one of the best antioxidants and anti-inflammatory supplements. It can be used for both heart protection and cancer prevention as well as for mental health. If you want more heart protection, have high cholesterol, or a family history of heart disease, use more EPA than DHA. The combined total of the marine oils EPA:DHA should be at least two grams per day. If you suffer from arthritis, lupus, or other rheumatic diseases, use about four grams per day. If you have a history of depression, ADHD, anxiety, or are planning on becoming pregnant, use DHA which helps with fetal brain development and can help improve mental well-being. If you are a vegetarian, use four grams of flaxseed oil.

Vitamin D is an important supplement for preventing osteoporosis and heart disease for women of all ages. You can use Vitamin D3 as well as spend fifteen to twenty minutes in the sun. Take about 1000 units of Vitamin D3 to maintain optimal levels.

FOR MEN

CoQ10 is important for your body's ability to produce energy. Use 100 mg daily, but if you are training for an endurance sport such as a marathon or have a chronic disease, use 300 mg/day because your body needs to produce more energy to keep up with your extra workouts and/or disease process.

L Carnitine works with CoQ10 to help the energy cycle work faster. It helps bring long-chain fatty acids into the cell for energy and helps remove toxins and waste from your cells. It can also help with exercise tolerance, improve heart function and energy, and decrease cholesterol. I recommend this for men after age 40 or earlier if you have a chronic disease.

Multivitamins must have about 5000 units of Vitamin A (to help with vision and skin renewal), calcium (1000 mg), magnesium (500 mg), trace amounts of selenium (for bone health), Vitamin E and C (good antioxidants, but you don't need to overdo them), and Vitamin B complex (for nerve health, mental health, and skin and hair health). I favor using a multivitamin because our hectic lives often prevent us from obtaining these in our daily lives. A good multivitamin can help.

Omega-3 fish oil is one of the best antioxidants and anti-inflammatory supplements for all men. The two marine components in fish oil are EPA and DHA. Combined together they should be over two grams per day to help decrease your cholesterol and reduce your risk of cancer, Alzheimer's, and hypertension. If you suffer from arthritis, lupus, or other rheumatic diseases, use about four grams per day. If you have a history of depression, ADHD, or anxiety, use DHA to help improve mental well-being. If you are a vegetarian, use four grams of flaxseed oil.

Prostate formula: Use a formula that has 200 mg of saw palmetto daily (which helps inhibit production of dihydrotestosterone, a breakdown product of testosterone that contributes to prostate enlargement); 100 mg of pygeum (a bark that lowers levels of inflammatory compounds in the prostate; when used in combination with saw palmetto, urinary flow improves); and 300 mg of nettle root (which research has shown to interact with dihydrotestosterone to possibly help improve sexual function).

Vitamin D is an important supplement for preventing osteoporosis and heart disease. You can use Vitamin D3 as well as spend fifty to twenty minutes in the sun. Take about 1000 units of Vitamin D3 to maintain optimal levels.

A Note on Supplements

Since supplements are not regulated by the FDA, many vitamins may contain less than 90 percent of the stated vitamin or mineral. There are three levels of vitamins:

Pharmaceutical Grade: means they have a pharmaceutical standard.

Food Grade: meets standard for human consumption.

Feed Grade: meets standard for animal consumption.

The differences between these levels are the quality and purity of vitamins. Always make sure you are using pharmaceutical grade supplements or they may not be effective and can cause other problems.

FLUIDS

The most important fluid is water. It is vital for us to keep hydrated with water. The chronic inflammation that comes from daily activity produces heat and dehydration, which can decrease fluid in our joints and cause our vertebral discs to dry out and shrink. Hydration prompts our bodies to make lubricating fluids. Most people walk around at least 1.5 liters per day underhydrated. You should try to drink one half ounce per pound you weigh. So if you weigh 150 pounds, drink 75 ounces of water per day.

Green tea is an excellent beverage. It can protect against cancers of the breast, prostate, esophagus, stomach, colon, lung, skin, liver, bladder, ovary, and blood (such as leukemia). Make sure you are drinking the real thing—not a green tea full of sugar!

EATING WELL IS A LIFESTYLE

Creating this spoke on your Personal Wellness Wheel™ is different from what you may have learned about nutrition. Eating well is a lifestyle choice and commitment. Periodic dieting is not the solution. You cannot diet for the rest of your life, but you can eat well. Also, if you noticed, I did not talk about calories. Calories are not as important as the glycemic index. I want you to eat a serving of a healthy protein and two good carbohydrates (most fruits, vegetables, or multigrain snacks) with every meal and one good carbohydrate or protein as a snack. Remember: a serving size is the size of your cupped palm.

But you don't have to be perfect. I tell everyone to build in "cheat days." Most Americans cheat every day. We rationalize that if we eat a little something bad, we can make up for it later. But it is better to have five days of no cheating followed by two days of some mild cheating. Or go three days without cheating and one day with. Look at your own schedule and see what works for you. But as often as possible, remember what you are doing this for: to look good, feel great, and live better!

THE MEDITERRANEAN DIET

Now it's time to put all this information together into a diet that will form this element of your Personal Wellness Wheel™. We will use what is known as a Mediterranean Diet which will help you:

❖ Reduce body fat
❖ Improve glucose and insulin utilization
❖ Lower blood pressure, total cholesterol, LDL cholesterol, and triglycerides
❖ Improve HDL cholesterol
❖ Improve overall endothelial (blood vessel wall) function
❖ Reduce inflammation at the cellular level

FOODS IN THE MEDITERRANEAN DIET

This diet includes all the principles we have discussed in this chapter. Specifically, it is made up of:

❖ Fruits and vegetables: at least seven servings per day (avoid melons, tropical fruits, potatoes, and corn)
❖ Fish (cold-water): three to four times per week
❖ Dairy: nonfat and low-fat in limited amounts only

❖ Eggs: up to four per week, preferably without the yolk
❖ Grains, legumes, and nuts: whole grain, fiber-rich cereals, breads, pastas. (If you are trying to lose weight, limit nuts and nut butters.)
❖ Plant proteins: at least one to two sources per day in the form of legumes, beans, soybeans, tofu, tempeh, or unsalted nuts.
❖ Meat: limit red meat to one to two times per month and consume mostly lean meats in limited quantities (e.g., chicken & turkey).
❖ Fiber: consume at least twenty-five to thirty-five grams per day.
❖ Virgin olive oil and canola oil
❖ Alcohol: limit intake to about one glass of red wine per day. Those who have difficulty with moderating alcohol, which is about 30 percent of all drinkers, should avoid all alcohol.

For your convenience and ease of reference, pages 69-70 have a grocery list that you can bring to the store with you. It lists good foods and also foods that you should limit (noted with ■) and foods that you should always avoid (noted with ⊠).

BUILDING SPOKE THREE
OF YOUR PERSONAL WELLNESS WHEEL™

Building and maintaining the third spoke is a life-long, daily task. Here are some tips to help you:

❑ Examine your eating patterns (that you learned about in Chapter Two) and target any unhealthy habits (e.g., bad-for-you comfort foods, eating when not hungry). Start to keep a food diary.

❑ Clean out your cupboards, work desk, or other hiding places; get rid of refined, processed foods. And don't buy more. (Bonus: these foods are usually also high in overt sugars and bad fats.)

❑ Start reading labels on your foods. Better yet, choose products with no labels—those that are found in nature!

❑ Be natural! Shop the perimeter of the grocery store—stock up on fruits, veggies, fish, and dairy.

❑ Start your day right: eat a low GI index, healthy breakfast (such as eggs with vegetables).

❑ Visit www.glycemicindex.com. Make a list of your favorite foods or foods you'd like to try that are low GI/low GL. Also make a list of high GI/GL foods to avoid or cut back on.

❑ Foods to avoid or cut back:
   ❖ Saturated fats: from animals or tropical oils (e.g., palm, coconut). Consume no more than a palm-size of meat or a tablespoon of these oils per day.
   ❖ Trans fats/hydrogenated oils: cut completely. Many foods with these products are now labeled.
   ❖ Corn, potatoes, melons, tropical fruits, and foods made from white flour or white rice.

❑ Eat these good fats:
   ❖ Monounsaturated fats: Try switching to olive or canola oil.
   ❖ Omega-3s: From cold-water fish, fish capsules, enriched eggs, soybeans, walnuts, and flaxseed.

❑ Add a handful of unsalted, unsweetened nuts to your diet every day.

❑ Eat at least thirty grams of fiber per day (from fruits, veggies, nuts, whole grains, and seeds).

❑ Expand your repertoire of whole grains—try quinoa, millet, kamut, or others.

❑ If you eat animal products, try to eat those that are grass-fed or organic. Start cutting back and replacing meat with organically-grown plant foods.

- ❑ Consume healthy proteins: chicken, turkey, fish, eggs, soy products, low-fat dairy.
- ❑ Add "super green" foods (wheat germ, barley, wheat grass, alfalfa, chlorella, spirulina, or blue-green algae) to your diet.
- ❑ Spice it up! Add spices to whatever you are eating.
- ❑ Use the supplements discussed. Be sure to read labels for information on quality and dosages.
- ❑ Drink water. Lots of it. Carry a water bottle.
- ❑ Drink green tea. Use it to replace something you now drink, such as coffee, black tea, or soda.
- ❑ Be careful when eating out, as restaurants often use unhealthy oils or ingredients you may not know about. You have more control at home. If you eat out, plan ahead. Bad decisions are made when you are hungry!
- ❑ Try the menu ideas on p. 56. Try out new foods or new combinations. Start with small changes.
- ❑ Don't think you have to completely give up foods you like but which aren't so great for you. Build in "cheat days" when you can eat these in moderation.
- ❑ Slow down! Enjoy what you eat.

GROCERY LIST
Good-for-you Choices

Proteins:

- White-meat, skinless chicken and turkey (grilled, baked, broiled, boiled, stir fried, sautéed)
- Cold-water fish: salmon, tuna, sardines, mackerel, steelhead trout
- Soy, tofu, edamame
- Beans
- Nuts
- Milk (skim or soy)
- Low-fat dairy (cheeses, yogurts)
- Eggs (preferably free-range, omega-3 enriched)

Carbohydrates:

❑ Fruits
- Apples, peaches, plums, nectarines, grapes, cherries, oranges, tangerines, grapefruits, strawberries, blueberries, blackberries, raspberries, pears, apricots

❑ Vegetables
- Super green foods: wheat germ, barley, alfalfa sprouts, wheat grass, sea algae, spirulina, chlorella, and green tea
- Tip: use vinagareitte dressing on salad.

❑ Multigrains
- Multigrain breads (with three to five grams of fiber per slice); good multigrain breads contain no sugar or sugar substitutes.
- Stone-ground, whole grain pasta
- High-fiber, whole grain cereal (All Bran®, Fiber One®, or Kashi Whole Grains, High Fiber)
- Oats, including old-fashioned oatmeal
- Whole wheat crackers (Triscuits are okay)

■ Millet	■ Rye
■ Barley	■ Quinoa
■ Brown Rice	■ Kamut

Fats:

❑ Good fats
- Omega-9s: olive oil, canola oil, and nuts (almonds, cashews, pistachios, macadamia, Brazilian nuts, peanuts)
- Omega-3s (soy, tofu, soybean, walnuts, cold water fish, flaxseed)

GROCERY LIST
FOODS TO LIMIT OR AVOID

Proteins:

- ■ Limit marine life such as shell fish (once per week)
- ■ Limit red meat (grass-fed, organic only once or twice per month)
- ■ Limit pork (rarely eat)
- ☒ Poultry skin
- ☒ Fast food or fatty meats
- ☒ Milk with bovine growth hormone or antibiotics
- ☒ Yellow or hard cheeses (they contain hydrogenated oils, artificial colors, and flavors)
- ☒ Cream and whipping cream
- ☒ Margarine
- ☒ Yogurt with aspartame (NutraSweet®)

Carbohydrates:

- ❑ Fruits
  - ☒ *Avoid tropical fruits (papaya, pineapple, mango, banana) and melons (watermelon, honeydew, and cantaloupe)*
- ❑ Vegetables
  - ☒ Avoid potatoes and corn
- ❑ Starches
  - ☒ Packaged goods with hydrogenated oils
  - ☒ Products made with white flour
  - ☒ Baked goods (pies, cookies, donuts, etc.)
  - ☒ Bread such as bagels, rolls, or croissants
  - ☒ Crackers and pretzels
  - ☒ Instant oatmeal
  - ☒ White pasta
  - ☒ Potatoes (white, red, instant)
  - ☒ White or instant rice or rice cakes

Fats:

- ☒ Saturated fats (animal fat, palm or coconut oil)
- ☒ Trans fats (solid at room temperature)
- ☒ Polyunsaturated omega-6s (corn, safflower, sunflower, cottonseed oils)
- ☒ Fried foods, lard, or shortening
- ☒ Hydrogenated/partially hydrogenated oils
- ☒ Peanut butter with added sugar or hydrogenated oils

MENU IDEAS FOR EATING WELL

Breakfast Options:

All options include eight ounces of water and green tea.

Old-fashioned or steel-cut oatmeal with fruits, nuts, and cinnamon

Cereal: Fiber One® Original, Kashi High Fiber with fruit and soy or skim milk

Eggs (any style) with fresh veggies such as spinach, broccoli, onions, tomatoes

Low-fat cottage cheese with fruits (berries, peaches, nectarines, apricots, apples)

Lean cut of ham and fruit or slices of tomatoes and cucumbers

Plain yogurt or Greek yogurt with fruit and nuts

Smoked salmon with fresh tomatoes, cucumbers, and fruit

Assorted low-fat cheeses, grapes, tomatoes

Lunch Options:

All options include eight ounces of water and green tea; add fruit for dessert.

Salad with chicken, tuna, salmon, or lots of beans; soup if needed

Fish or chicken breast with two sides of vegetables

Open-faced lean turkey or ham sandwich on wheat bread with lots of veggies

Shrimp or chicken stirfry with brown rice

Sushi made with brown rice

Tofu burger or open-faced grilled chicken or turkey burger

Dinner Options:

All options include eight ounces of water and green tea; include one green vegetable with each entrée; if you need a grain, try brown rice, kamut, barley, whole wheat couscous, quinoa, or whole wheat pasta.

Grilled fish or chicken with two vegetables

Baked turkey, fish, or chicken with two vegetables and a grain

Shrimp, chicken, or vegetable stirfry with brown rice

Stovetop chicken, turkey, or bean stews

Chicken kabobs

Chili (vegetarian, turkey, or occasionally beef)

Whole wheat pasta with turkey or occasionally with beef

Whole wheat pizza with low-fat mozzarella cheese, loaded with fresh veggies

Snack Options:

Handful of unsalted nuts and a piece of fruit

Turkey slices, low-fat cheese, and grape tomatoes or other vegetables

Hummus or baba ganoush with carrots, celery, cucumbers, or 1/2 whole wheat pita

Slices of green and red peppers or other veggies with low-fat cheese

Yogurt with nuts or seeds

Multigrain bread or apple with all-natural peanut, almond, or cashew butter

Protein bar

DIET HISTORY

Use the following Diet History Form for a week. See what your usual food choices are and compare with the choices provided in this chapter to see where you need to make changes. You can create your own menu from the choices provided or based on the information in the Mediterranean Diet or sign up for our weekly meal planner by email to help structure your week and grocery shopping.

	Breakfast	Snack	Lunch	Snack	Dinner	Snack
S U N D						
M O N D						
T U E S D						
W E D N E S						
T H U R S D						
F R I D						
S A T U R						

THE POWER OF EXERCISE: MAINTAINING A YOUTHFUL MIND AND BODY

To be idle is a short road to death and to be diligent is a way of life; foolish people are idle, wise people are diligent.

~ Buddha

We need to integrate our breathing, flexibility, coordination, and muscle tone to help slow the degenerative process. In the

modern world most of us sit throughout the day, adding weight and losing muscle mass with each passing year. We rarely connect our mind and body together in our daily activities. Most of us are not conscious of our breathing patterns or how we are losing our natural agility with age. This spoke of the Personal Wellness Wheel™ will help create a holistic exercise program that will slow aging by working on the mind and body together. Optimal Health is the continuous balance of the mind, body, and spirit.

In this chapter, you will learn the following:
○ Why Exercise is so Important
○ Types of Physical Exercise
○ Importance of Breathing
○ Fitness Plan Levels

WHY EXERCISE IS SO IMPORTANT

Your body receives only two messages: grow or decay. You have a choice; you decide every day which message you are sending. Exercise connects the mind and body together with your breathing which is one of the strongest signals your body receives to foster growth.

BODY MASS INDEX

As we age, we lose muscle mass and increase our body fat. The loss of muscle mass is called sarcopenia. We begin to lose muscle mass after the age of 24, losing about 1.4 percent per year. This loss means that by the time we are age 50, we will have lost almost 30 percent of our muscle mass.

Women have more body fat than men because women bear children. In order for a woman to have regular menstrual cycles, she should have at least 17-18 percent body fat. Having less than this can cause menstrual irregularities and bone loss. Ideally women should be around 20 percent body fat. Men should aim for about 10 percent.

Body mass index (BMI) is a number calculated from your height and weight and is an important measure of health. To calculate your BMI, use the formula: weight (in pounds) / [height (in inches squared)] x 703. Let's calculate your BMI and see where you fit it. Take your weight, divide it by your height in inches squared and then multiply the whole amount by 703. For example if your weight is 150 pounds and your height is

5'5" (you are 65" tall), the calculation would be [150 ÷ (65)^2] x 703 = 24.96

Now to find out if you are have a healthy BMI, refer to the chart below or visit our Website at www.optimalhealthtoday.com.

BMI	Weight Status
Below 18.5	Underweight
18.5 – 24.9	Normal
25.0 – 29.9	Overweight
30.0 and above	Obese

PHYSICAL BENEFITS OF EXERCISE

Benefits for the Heart

Exercise can improve cardiovascular health. The *Archives of Internal Medicine* in January 2008 showed an increased risk of non-fatal cardiovascular events and mortality in those who had a diminished exercise capacity when they were put through an exercise stress test. That means the less exercise you do, the greater your risk for having a heart problem!

A study in the *British Journal of Sports Medicine* in 2008 talked about how diminished or slowed aerobic fitness was associated with the loss of independent living for older seniors. Aerobic capacity begins to decline during middle age and continues as we get older. A gentle aerobic program can improve your aerobic capacity and your chances of living independently as you age.

Improving Diabetes and Metabolic Syndrome

People who exercise regularly are less likely to develop diabetes than people who do not. Exercise improves blood glucose control by improving cardiovascular health and building muscle, which decreases insulin resistance. The *Annals of Internal Medicine* stated that the best method exercise to help reduce blood glucose levels in diabetics is combining both aerobic and weight training. (Please see page 76 for a description of metabolic syndrome.)

Improving Longevity with Exercise

The Framingham study (which studied over 5000 people for forty-six years) found that of the people who reached age 50, those who exercised lived on average 4.6 years longer! Just with exercise we can live longer!

In another study, researchers examined whether people who exercised regularly had longer telomere lengths. Telomeres are fragments of DNA that serve as an impor-

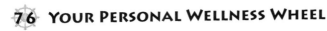

tant part of cell replication. With time, telomeres begin to degenerate from natural oxidative stress and inflammation in the body. Researchers found that people who smoked and had a sedentary lifestyle had shorter telomere lengths. This is an important message that even when our bodies begin to degenerate, exercise is a powerful anti-aging tool!

Reducing the Risk of Cancer

Obesity and physical inactivity also increase cancer risk. In 2001, the National Institutes of Health concluded that cancers of the colon, breast (postmenopausal), endometrium (the uterine lining), kidney, and esophagus are associated with obesity. Some studies have also reported links between obesity and cancers of the gallbladder, ovaries, and pancreas. Preventing weight gain can reduce the risk of many cancers. Experts recommend that people establish habits of healthy eating and physical activity early in life to prevent becoming overweight or obese. Those who are already overweight or obese are advised to avoid additional weight gain and to lose weight through a low-calorie diet and exercise. Even a weight loss of only 5 to 10 percent of total weight can provide health benefits.

Reducing the Risk of Colon Cancer

The BBC in 2001 reported that a review of fifty different studies found that people who exercised regularly halved their risk of colon cancer! Along with exercise, these participants also ate a healthy diet full of vegetables and fruits.

In the *American Journal of Epidemiology*, researchers found that both men and women lowered their risk of colorectal cancer with physical activity. Men and women who exercised an amount equivalent to jogging five or more hours per week lowered their risk of colorectal cancer by 40 to 50 percent. Some benefit came from less vigorous activity, particularly for rectal cancer.

Reducing the Risk of Prostate Cancer

In a prospective study done in Norway, researchers found that regular exercise decreased the risk of advanced prostate cancer and overall cancer death.

Reducing the Risk of Breast Cancer

The California Teachers study that evaluated women between 20-79 years of age from 1995-2002 who did not have breast cancer found that strenuous regular exercise was a powerful protective effect against breast cancer. The Iowa Women's Health Study of postmenopausal women found that regular exercise decreased the risk of breast cancer. This sends a powerful message to women with a family history of breast cancer and to women in general that exercising can decrease the risk for one of the most common cancers women can get.

Exercise and Memory

A 2003 CNN report discussed how exercise helps improve memory. People who regularly exercise are less likely to lose muscle function, including the brain. MRI scans done on volunteers showed that people who exercised had greater gray matter than people who did not exercise.

Exercise and Mood

Exercise can help improve emotional states such as depression, anxiety, and over-all mood. A review of different studies done in Poland showed that aerobic activity for fifteen to thirty minutes per day three times per week was associated with reduced anxiety and depression.

Exercise and Brain Function

Exercise improves what scientists call "executive function," the set of skills and abilities that allow you to choose appropriate behavior for a situation and to focus on the job at hand. These skills include memory, response, and processing speed.

Executive function starts to decline when people reach their 70s. But elderly people who have been athletic all their lives have much better executive function than sedentary people of the same age. When inactive people get more exercise, even starting in their 70s, their executive function improves.

Exercise is also strongly associated with a reduced risk of dementia late in life. People who exercise regularly in middle age are one-third as likely to get Alzheimer's disease in their 70s as those who did not exercise. Even people who begin exercising in their 60s can still reduce their risk of dementia.

How does exercise help the brain? Fitness training slows the age-related shrink-age of the frontal cortex, which is important for executive function. Exercise may also help the brain by improving cardiovascular health and preventing heart attacks and small strokes that can cause brain damage, also referred to as multi-infarct dementia. Finally, exercise causes the release of growth factors (proteins that increase the num-ber of connections between neurons) and the birth of neurons in the hippocampus (a brain region important for memory).

TYPES OF PHYSICAL EXERCISE

Now that we know how important exercise is, let's examine the types of physical exercise that will benefit you. Again, not all types of exercise are good for everyone. An exercise regimen needs to be customized based upon your initial condition, age, medical conditions, and goals. Remember to always consult your physician prior to beginning an exercise program.

AEROBIC EXERCISE

Aerobic exercise is any exercise that requires the heart and lungs to work harder to meet the body's need for oxygen. Aerobic exercise is beneficial because it

- ❖ reduces the risk of obesity, heart disease, high blood pressure, type 2 diabetes, stroke, and certain types of cancer.
- ❖ helps lower blood pressure.
- ❖ improves insulin sensitivity and blood glucose control.
- ❖ reduces arthritis and chronic muscle pain.
- ❖ helps you lose weight when combined with a healthy diet.
- ❖ helps improve your immune system so you are less likely to become sick.
- ❖ increases HDL ("good") cholesterol and decreases LDL ("bad") cholesterol.
- ❖ strengthens your heart so it pumps more effectively and efficiently.
- ❖ helps boost your mood and reduces anxiety and stress.
- ❖ increases your stamina and endurance. (You may be tired right after exercising, but with time your body becomes stronger so that it won't become fatigued.)
- ❖ helps maintain your cognitive skills and reduces the risk of dementia.
- ❖ reduces silent inflammation.
- ❖ reduces resting heart rate.
- ❖ may help you live longer.

Types of Aerobic Activities:		
❖ running	❖ biking	❖ dancing
❖ jumping	❖ elliptical	❖ stair climbing
❖ swimming	❖ cross country skiing	❖ rowing

ANAEROBIC EXERCISE

Anaerobic exercises are very short, intense activities in which the body runs out of oxygen and begins to get its energy by breaking down fat cells. Examples are heavy weight-lifting, sprints (running, biking, etc.), jumping rope, hill climbing, interval training, isometrics (in which one part of the body is used to resist the movement of another part), or any rapid burst of hard exercise.

Anaerobic exercise is beneficial because it

❖ develops stronger muscles.

❖ improves heart and lungs because it forces the building of new capillaries to increase oxygen. (Your body can begin to tolerate greater lactic acid build-up, a byproduct of anaerobic exercise. It is what makes you feel achy the next day. When done regularly, your body is able to clear it faster which improves your endurance in the long run.)

❖ increases your basal metabolism rate.

❖ increases muscle mass and bone mass.

❖ makes you faster.

❖ decreases body fat.

❖ helps you release more growth hormone.

There are two types of anaerobic training: resistance training and interval training.

Resistance Training

Resistance training is any exercise that causes the muscles to contract against something (such as dumbbells, rubber exercise tubing, or your own body weight). Resistance training works by causing microscopic damage or tears to the muscle cells, which in turn are quickly repaired by the body to help the muscles regenerate and grow stronger. Muscles heal and grow when you aren't working out; that is why it's necessary to leave time between workouts for recovery.

Warning: If you do not do resistance training, you will lose muscle, which results in flab and fat. As we age, we lose muscle. Up to age 50, people lose about 4 percent of their strength and muscle mass per decade. After that, the loss increases to about 10 percent per decade. By age 60 the average man and woman will have lost about one-third of their muscle mass . . . unless they make an effort to reverse this process through exercise.

Types of Resistance Training:
❖ Free Weights
❖ Machines
❖ Exercise Tubing

Interval Training

Interval training is a great anaerobic exercise. It can be done with many types of exercise (for example, running, biking, or swimming). An interval is done by increasing your pace as fast as you can for one to two minutes and then coming to a very slow walk or stop. You need to recover, get your heart rate below 110, and then burst out again for one to two minutes. You repeat this about eight times, always trying to stay at the same speed at which you started. This is hard and very tiring. You must come to a rest because this helps you build those fast-twitch muscle fibers that you are beginning to lose with age and helps your speed. If you can only do four repetitions in the beginning, just do four. I would rather have you do it well than cheat.

CAUTION: Anaerobic interval training is ONLY for those who are very fit and desire to increase speed, lactate threshold, and overall aerobic power.

FLEXIBILITY AND BALANCE

Flexibility and balance are important and are especially helpful in combating stiffness associated with aging. Any of the below methods can help, but I am partial to yoga. Yoga means union. It is the union of the mind and body through breath. It is meditation in motion. Yoga is one of the most complete exercises we can do because it incorporates breathing, flexibility, balance, and resistance training (using your body weight). Yoga can be part of your regular exercise schedule or can be done by itself. Even if only done once per week, it will help balance your mind, body, and spirit.

Improving Your Flexibility and Balance:
❖ Tai Chi
❖ Yoga
❖ Stretching
❖ Dancing

IMPORTANCE OF BREATHING

Breathing is one of the most instinctive things we do. In the traditional Indian medicine of Aryurveda, the breath is called *prana*, the vital energy that nourishes the body and soul. Without *prana*, all of us would die. The deeper and more full our breathing is, the greater nourishment we bring to our bodies.

The science of breathing called Pranayama is about integrating the mind and body.

Our breath mirrors our soul. So, for example, when we are scared, our breathing is faster and more shallow. When we become more relaxed, our breathing becomes deeper and fuller. Most of the time we are not conscious of breathing, but during exercise you can focus on this. Yoga is the easiest exercise to do this with, but you can be conscious of your breathing with any exercise. This new awareness of breath can be applied throughout the day to help you integrate and balance your mind and body. You will learn more about breathing in the stress management section (Chapter Seven).

BUILDING SPOKE FOUR
OF YOUR PERSONAL WELLNESS WHEEL™

Now let's build the fourth spoke of the wheel with your exercise plan:

❑ If you have not exercised before, start slowly!

❑ First, let's test your **heart rate**. This is a quick test to see how physically fit you are. Count your pulse at rest for one minute while sitting quietly and again first thing in the morning before you even get up. Typically, the slower your heart is the better shape you are in. If your heart rate is too slow (below 50) it can suggest other problems, but athletic individuals can have a low resting heart rate because they are in great shape. If you are not in great shape, you need to see someone!

Great condition: heart rate below 60 resting
Good condition: heart rate between 60-70
Need to start exercising more: 71-80
Need to exercise, period! Above 81
Above 90: Too high; consult your physician because something may be going on.

Why is your resting heart rate important? Your heart is a machine. The more work it has to do, the faster it will wear down. But isn't exercise more work? No, because while exercise momentarily increases your heart's work, over time, your heart gets stronger so each time it contracts, it can pump out even more blood. Thus, it can do less work and be more effective. The higher your pulse rate, the more work your heart has to do, and the faster it begins to wear down. Along with the other problems it begins to face hardening arteriole walls and increased blood pressure. Help your heart out and start exercising!

❑ Next, determine your **age group** and use the following general exercise guide:

Age 40 or younger: 50% aerobic, 25% strength, and 25% yoga
Age 41 to 50: 40% aerobic, 30% strength, and 30% yoga
Age 51 and older: 30% aerobic, 30% strength ,and 30% yoga

If you are above age 40, consult your physician prior to starting an exercise program. If you are beginning a program and are over age 40 or have a chronic medical condition such as diabetes, you should have a stress test. Once you have your doctor's permission, start slowly. Below is a general guideline for various exercise plans. Once you are stronger you can move to the next level (in about eight to ten weeks). To customize your program, consider a personal trainer.

Fitness Level	
Never exercised:	Begin with walking program
Exercise 1-2 times per week:	Level one program-beginning
Exercise 3-4 times per week:	Level two program-intermediate
Exercise 5 or more times per week:	Level three program-advanced

FITNESS PLAN: BEGINNING WALKING

TRAINING LOG   DATES:

WORKOUT	TRAINING PLAN	Mon	Tues	Wed	Thu	Fri	Sat	Sun
10 minutes Stretching	Four times per week after walking							
Walking	Fast pace for 30 minutes one time per week							
Walking	On an incline for 30 minutes one time per week							
Walking	Moderate pace for 45 minutes one time per week							
Walking	Slower pace for 60 minutes one time per week							
Abdominal Exercises (20 of each type)	10 min: four times per week Reverse crunches							
	Forward crunches							
	Oblique crunches							
Total number of workout hours								4 hours

FITNESS PLAN: LEVEL ONE TRAINING LOG

WORK-OUT	TRAINING PLAN	Mon	Tues	Wed	Thu	Fri	Sat	Sun
Stretching	10 min, at least four times per week							
Cardio	30 minutes, two times per week							
Yoga	45-60 min per week							
Abdominal Exercises (30 of each type)	10 min: four times per week Reverse crunches							
	Forward crunches							
	Oblique crunches							
Weight Training	Area targeted two times per week (30 min)							
Chest	Bench Press (2 sets/ 10 reps)							
	Incline Press (2 sets/ 10 reps)							
Back	Lateral Pulldown (2 sets/ 10 reps)							
	Cable Rows (2 sets/10 reps)							
Squats	Feet straight (2 sets/10 reps)							
	Feet turned out (2 sets/ 10 reps)							
Lunges	Forward lunge (2 sets/10 reps)							
	Reverse lunge (2 sets/ 10 reps)							

FITNESS PLAN: LEVEL TWO TRAINING LOG

WORK-OUT	TRAINING PLAN	Mon	Tues	Wed	Thu	Fri	Sat	Sun
Stretch-ing	10 min, four times per week							
Cardio	30 minutes, one time per week							
Yoga	45-60 min per week							
Sprinting	20 min, one time per week 6 times, 100 yard dash							
Abdomi-nal Exercises (30 of each type)	10 min: four times per week Reverse crunches Forward crunches Oblique crunches							
Weight Training	Area targeted two times per week (30 min)							
Chest	Bench Press (2 sets/ 10 reps) Incline Press (2 sets/ 10 reps)							
Back	Lateral Pulldown (2 sets/ 10 reps) Cable Rows (2 sets/10 reps)							
Squats	Feet straight (2 sets/10 reps) Feet turned out (2 sets/ 10 reps)							
Lunges	Forward lunge (2 sets/10 reps) Reverse lunge (2 sets/ 10 reps)							

FITNESS PLAN: LEVEL THREE TRAINING LOG

WORK-OUT	TRAINING PLAN	Mon	Tues	Wed	Thu	Fri	Sat	Sun
Stretching	10 min, four times per week							
Cardio	30 minutes, two times per week							
Yoga	60 min per week							
Sprinting	20 min, two times per week 8 times, 100 yard dash							
Abdominal Exercises (30 of each type)	10 min: four times per week Reverse crunches							
	Forward crunches							
	Oblique crunches							
Weight Training	Area targeted two times per week (45 min)							
Chest	Bench Press (3 sets/ 10 reps)							
	Incline Press (3 sets/ 10 reps)							
Back	Lateral Pulldown (3 sets/ 10 reps)							
	Cable Rows (3 sets/10 reps)							
Squats	Feet straight (3 sets/10 reps)							
	Feet turned out (3 sets/ 10 reps)							
Lunges	Forward lunge (3 sets/10 reps)							
	Reverse lunge (3 sets/ 10 reps)							

FITNESS PLAN: LEVEL FOUR TRAINING LOG

WORK-OUT	TRAINING PLAN	Mon	Tues	Wed	Thu	Fri	Sat	Sun
Stretch-ing	10 min, four times per week							
Cardio	30 minutes, two times per week							
Yoga	60 min, two times per week							
Sprinting	20 min, two time per week 10 times, 100 yard dash							
Abdomi-nal Exercises (30 of each type)	10 min: four times per week Reverse crunches Forward crunches Oblique crunches							
Weight Training	Area targeted two times per week (45 min)							
Chest	Bench Press (3 sets/ 10 reps) Incline Press (3 sets/ 10 reps)							
Back	Lateral Pulldown (3 sets/ 10 reps) Cable Rows (3 sets/10 reps)							
Squats	Feet straight (3 sets/10 reps) Feet turned out (3 sets/ 10 reps)							
Lunges	Forward lunge (3 sets/10 reps) Reverse lunge (3 sets/ 10 reps)							

❏ Keep track of your Body Mass Index (see page 75).
❏ Exercise Guide:
- ❖ For strength training, use free weights, machines, or exercise tubing. Only the most important muscle groups are included in the exercise templates in the previous pages. Change your routine by adding weights or trying a new exercise every six to eight weeks.
- ❖ Warm your body up and then stretch before and after exercise. Yoga can be part of your stretching routine if you cannot do it separately.
- ❖ Be conscious of your breathing.
- ❖ Don't exercise if it causes pain. Pain is a sign of an injury.
- ❖ For better workouts, get a personal trainer.
- ❖ Please visit our Website's personal training section to learn more about how to perform these exercises.

SUMMARY OF EXERCISE BENEFITS

- ❖ Controls body fat
- ❖ Prevents degenerative diseases
- ❖ Reduces risk for breast and colon cancer
- ❖ Enhances self-image
- ❖ Elevates mood
- ❖ Reduces stress
- ❖ Improves appearance
- ❖ Increases energy
- ❖ Enhances feeling of well-being
- ❖ Reinforces healthier eating habits
- ❖ Stimulates creative thinking
- ❖ Restores function to organs, muscles, joints, and bones
- ❖ Improves healing
- ❖ Reduces low-grade inflammation
- ❖ Improves insulin sensitivity

YOUR GUIDE TO HORMONE OPTIMIZATION: RESTORING YOUR BODY'S BALANCE

What lies behind us and what lies before us are tiny matters compared to what lies within us.

~ Oliver Wendell Holmes

CONTENTS:

This chapter will help you learn about the benefits and risks of hormone therapy, as well as educate you about hormones and their importance. Hormone therapy is controversial, and research continues on how therapies affect us. This decision must not be made lightly; it requires that you educate yourself thoroughly and consult a qualified physician or Age Management Specialist to make an informed decision.

I have included many clinical references in this chapter because I want you to be able to read the clinical studies if you wish. I have also included references in the appendix for more information.

In this chapter, you will learn the following:

- ❍ The Importance and Function of Hormones
- ❍ Testosterone for Men
- ❍ Menopause
- ❍ Hormone Replacement for Women
- ❍ DHEA
- ❍ Thyroid Hormone
- ❍ Human Growth Hormone

THE IMPORTANCE AND FUNCTION OF HORMONES

Hormone loss is one of the most important occurrences in the aging process. Age Management Specialists believe that good hormone health is important in slowing the process of aging and for increasing Optimal Health. Hormones help us maintain our internal balance by sending signals from the brain to the various parts of the body to control just about everything: growth, reproductive and sexual health, blood pressure, our desire to eat, food digestion, metabolism rate, bone and muscle structure. Critical hormones that help modulate the aging process for both men and women are testosterone, DHEA, thyroid hormone, and human growth hormone, as well as estrogen and progesterone in particular for women. Hormones that accelerate the aging process are insulin, which we discussed in the nutrition spoke (please see pages 57-58), and cortisol, the stress hormone, discussed in the stress management spoke (Chapter Seven).

As we age, starting in our 30s, we begin to lose about 1-3 percent of our critical hormones per year. This means that at the end of that decade, you may have lost 10-30 percent of your critical hormones. As these hormone levels diminish, you may feel vague symptoms of decreased energy, early fatigue, difficulty focusing or concentrating, lowered libido, and a greater plateau when exercising.

Optimizing your hormone health can lead to increased energy levels—including sexual energy, reduced body fat, and increased lean muscle. Improvements can also include better cognitive function, lower cholesterol, an enhanced mood, an improved ability to handle stress, and a stronger and more competent immune system, allowing you to remain as disease-free as possible. Each of these improvements enables your body to ward off chronic disease more successfully.

The goal in helping you achieve Optimal Health is to reduce the rate of these "normal" age-related declines so that you can maintain a healthy and productive life. Multiple studies have confirmed that our greatest fear as we age is losing our independence as a result of the onset and progressive worsening of chronic disease. Optimal Health aims to extend the independent, high quality period of your life.

Hormonal evaluation is an important part of the Optimal Health Program; it works in concert with the other spokes on your wheel. The following information will help you understand what symptoms might indicate that you could benefit from optimizing your hormones and the risks and benefits of the various hormones. Understanding these basic issues is important if you are contemplating a hormone replacement program. I strongly recommend seeing an Age Management or hormone specialist to evaluate your situation. (Please visit our Website at www.optimalhealthtoday.com to get more information and learn about options for hormone replacement therapy.) Like any other important choice, a good decision is facilitated by doing your homework. We all need significant education and understanding when considering hormone replacement because everyone is NOT a candidate.

TESTOSTERONE FOR MEN

As research has shown, testosterone is a critical hormone for maintaining men's health. Testosterone receptor sites are found throughout the body. In the brain, testosterone helps with focus, concentration, memory, and improved mood. In the skeletal system, testosterone helps with building both muscle and bone mass. In the heart, it helps maintain proper function and regulate blood pressure. And of course, it helps improve libido and fertility.

After about age thirty to forty, men begin to lose about 1-3 percent of their testosterone per year (Feldmen, 2002). This begins a slow, steady decline for men (rather than the complete cessation of hormone production that occurs with women's menopause). This testosterone decline is called andropause or referred to as "male menopause." Because men's testosterone levels slowly decline, the symptoms of low testosterone can often be vague and non-specific, and the age at which they occur can vary.

Some men experience a faster decline. Men with chronic disease may have a greater chance of lower testosterone levels; men with illnesses such as diabetes, a history of heart attack or stroke, chronic liver disease, chronic kidney disease, chronic bronchitis or emphysema, HIV/AIDS, rheumatoid arthritis, obesity, cancer, traumatic brain injuries, burns, and chronic narcotic use are more likely to experience a testosterone deficiency (Kalyani, 2007).

Common symptoms men experience are a decrease in libido, erectile dysfunction, depression, irritability, and reduced memory, focus, and concentration as well as a diminished sense of well-being (Kalyani, 2007, Morales, 2002). The physical signs of low testosterone include muscle loss, bone mass loss, an increase in body fat (especially around the waist, hips, and buttocks), and a greater likelihood of developing male breasts (Becker, 2001; Kalyani, 2007; Morales, 2002).

ARE YOU AT RISK FOR LOW TESTOSTERONE? TAKE THE QUIZ.

To see if you are at risk for low testosterone, answer "yes" or "no" to the following questions. If you answer "yes" to question 1 or 7, or at least three of the other questions, you may have low testosterone. Be sure to discuss the results of this quiz with your doctor.

Choose the responses below that best describe how you have been feeling.

1. Do you have a decrease in libido (sex drive)?	Yes	No
2. Do you have a lack of energy?	Yes	No
3. Do you have a decrease in strength and/or endurance?	Yes	No
4. Have you lost height?	Yes	No
5. Have you noticed a decreased "enjoyment of life?"	Yes	No
6. Are you sad and/or grumpy?	Yes	No
7. Are your erections less strong?	Yes	No
8. Have you noticed a recent deterioration in your ability to play sports?	Yes	No
9. Are you falling asleep after dinner?	Yes	No
10. Has there been a recent deterioration in your work performance?	Yes	No

Source: Saint Louis University Androgen Deficiency in Aging Men (ADAM) Questionnaire. John Morley, M.D., Saint Louis University School of Medicine, June 1997.

If you answered yes to questions 1-7, you may be at risk for low testosterone and should consider getting your level checked.

Many of the above symptoms occur with what is perceived to be the "normal" course of aging. Distinguishing the cause of these general symptoms may require a little detective work by you and your physician. In fact, I now realize that some of the complaints from patients that I was unable to diagnose and treat early in my career were probably related to some hormonal imbalance. When nutrition, exercise, preventative medicine, and, if indicated, hormone replacement are optimized, you can slow the degenerative process.

Decreased hormones can cause serious health problems. As testosterone levels diminish, men lose muscle mass and increase body fat, especially around their midsections. This increased fat, also called visceral fat, increases their risk for insulin resistance, metabolic syndrome, diabetes, and heart disease. Metabolic syndrome is the complex of increased waist size, hypertension, elevated fasting blood sugar, and decreased HDL cholesterol. The presence of these factors increases an individual's risk of heart disease. As muscle mass declines, bones begin to thin, which increases the risk of falling and fractures. And while men are often overlooked in osteoporosis screening, one out of four men will develop osteoporosis (NIH, 2007). Heart disease, diabetes, and osteoporosis are unfortunately all too common in our aging population. These conditions are root causes of a potential decrease in our quality of life and loss of independence.

Preventing these changes does not occur by good fortune. It requires recognizing your individual changes and creating a customized, strategic plan of management like the Optimal Health Program. In this case, the old adage that "hope is not a plan" is particularly relevant.

Symptoms, along with measured testosterone levels, will help guide physicians in deciding whether testosterone therapy is appropriate. In older men, symptoms can be more indicative of low testosterone levels than actual blood levels (Araujo, 2007). Many people recommend checking saliva, but the "gold standard" (i.e., diagnostic method) is through blood work. If you are experiencing symptoms such as those on the previous page, you should consider checking your lab values. This is not part of a routine screening done by your primary care physician. You can ask your current physician if she or he will help you with this process, or you can seek out an Age Management physician who specializes in bio-identical hormone replacement (see page 100 for the difference between synthetic and bio-identical hormones).

If your levels are low, you may be a candidate for testosterone replacement. Testosterone replacement has been used successfully for the past fifteen years. Whether you are a candidate will depend on your symptoms, physical exams, and blood work as well as any other medical conditions that can interfere with testosterone therapy.

PSA

One of the most important tests your doctor will run to help determine whether you are a candidate for replacement is the PSA. What is this? Prostate-specific antigen (PSA) is a protein produced by the cells of the prostate gland. It is normal for men to have low PSA levels. Prostate cancer or benign (not cancerous) conditions such as inflammation of the prostate gland (prostatitis) or an enlargement of the prostate gland (benign prostatic hypertrophy, BPH) can increase PSA levels. The latter two do not cause cancer, but it is possible to have one or both of these conditions and develop prostate cancer as well.

The PSA test, along with a digital rectal exam (DRE), is the best way to detect prostate cancer in men. Ten percent of all men who have prostate cancer have a normal PSA; that is why the DRE is an essential component in men's health.

The risk factors for developing prostate cancer are being over 65 years of age, a family history of prostate cancer, being African American, and possibly a high-fat diet. Screening begins at age 40 or earlier if you are considering hormone replacement therapy.

Normal PSA levels are between 0.4-4 ng/ml. Optimal levels of the PSA are 0 to 2.5 ng/ml. Above 2.5 ng/ml, I recommend a urological evaluation prior to considering hormone replacement. Recent literature suggests that younger men with a PSA level greater than 2.5 ng/ml are at greater risk for developing prostate cancer. Know what your PSA level is because its trend can help detect early concerns. A one point increase in your PSA over one year merits further evaluation in our Optimal Health Program. A urologist needs to evaluate any PSA above 4.

The limitation of the PSA test is that it can only detect small, slow-growing tumors and not the aggressive tumors that can increase your risk of metastatic disease and death. Please always discuss your particular circumstances, the findings of this test, and the digital rectal exam with your physician.

TYPES OF REPLACEMENT

Testosterone replacement comes in various forms. You can use creams, gels, pellets, or injections. Your physician will discuss with you the best form for you.

COMMON SIDE EFFECTS OF TESTOSTERONE THERAPY

Some common side effects of testosterone therapy (when your levels become high) are mood swings, irritability, worsening of your cholesterol profile, acne, unwanted hair, and an increase in your red blood cells (which can cause blockages if you have narrow vessels). It is essential that you commit to a vigilant monitoring regimen to guide your dosing, especially in the beginning. Visits to your physician may be less frequent as your proper dosing is determined. It is also important for you to recognize and discuss with your physician any side effects you experience.

MENOPAUSE

As our society ages, more women will be living one-third to maybe even one-half their lives in the state of menopause! Ensuring that women have the best possible health in their postmenopausal years is an important step in Optimal Health.

Historically, menopause has been viewed as a dreaded time of life, characterized in the media and satirized in movies as a period filled with uncontrollable emotional outbursts, energy loss, and a series of undesirable behaviors. This is juxtaposed with portrayals of the male aging process, in which men are still virile and attractive. Yet menopause does not signal the end of a productive and happy life, but rather a new beginning for women and their lifecycles.

Menopause refers to a natural cessation in a woman's menstrual period and fertility. Menopause happens because the ovaries stop producing the hormones estrogen and progesterone. All women go through menopause, usually between the ages of 40 and 55. A woman has reached menopause when she has gone twelve months without having a period. Menopause can occur earlier if a woman has had premature ovarian failure or her ovaries surgically removed because she no longer produces estrogen and progesterone.

Menopausal symptoms can begin several years before in a stage called peri-menopause. Menopause and peri-menopause affect every woman differently, and the length of time each woman is symptomatic may vary from two to several years. Almost 85 percent of women experience some menopausal symptoms, some more disabling than others. A decrease in estrogen can affect many areas of the body including the genital area, the urinary system, the brain, the skin and hair, the skeleton, and the cardiovascular system.

CHANGES

Genito-Urinary System

As hormone levels decrease, the walls of the vagina become thinner, dryer, less elastic, and more susceptible to infection. This may also make intercourse uncomfortable. Tissues in the urinary tract also change and can cause incontinence and an increased susceptibility to urinary tract infection.

Menstrual Periods

Periods may be shorter or longer, heavier or lighter, or have more or less time between them. This occurs due to the fluctuating levels of hormones in the body. For chronic heavy bleeding and/or spotting, you should see your physician to confirm there are no other problems. You may also have breast pain.

Loss of Libido

A loss of libido may occur during and after menopause. Women have about one-tenth the testosterone levels that men have. The waning of premenopausal testosterone levels can contribute to a woman's loss of desire for sexual intercourse.

Neurological Symptoms

As hormone levels wane and fluctuate, women can experience different neurological symptoms such as
 ❖ Memory loss
 ❖ Difficulty concentrating (feeling like you are in a fog)
 ❖ Decreased attention
 ❖ Headaches
 ❖ Dizziness
 ❖ Fatigue
 ❖ Low energy levels
 ❖ Loss of vitality
 ❖ Weight gain
 ❖ Hot flashes
 ❖ Night sweats or cold sweats
 ❖ Trouble sleeping through the night.

Mental Health Changes

Mood swings, anxiety, irritability, and depression are sometimes associated with menopause. Estrogen therapy improves mood and dysphoria, possibly by affecting the metabolism of serotonin in the central nervous system (Sherwin, 1996). Depression in menopause is usually caused by other factors such as a woman's personal psychology, stress, or history of depression. Estrogen therapy can improve depression, but it does not help primary depression, which is a chemical imbalance in the brain (Cutson, 2006).

Skin and Hair Changes

Skin and hair changes associated with menopause include an increase in wrinkles and skin sagging, especially around the neck and jaw line. As the body ages, so does the skin. A dramatic decrease in collagen production during menopause may cause more wrinkles; collagen decreases by about 2.4 percent per year after menopause, double the loss of collagen and elastin a woman experiences in her 30s. So women are correct when they say they appear to be aging faster after menopause (Chung, 2004).

Unwanted facial hair is a common problem experienced during menopause. It comes from the change in estrogen and testosterone ratios in the body. Young women have very high levels of estrogen to testosterone. As women age, the estrogen to testosterone ratio becomes more equal, and women are more likely to experience unwanted facial hair. An Oxford study of 230 women found that women receiving hormone replacement had less facial hair than women who did not. However, that same study did not find that hormone replacement helped women with female pattern hair loss (Eedy, 2006).

A change in hair texture and the loss or thinning of hair can also occur with menopause; if they exist already, they may become worse. Treatment is complex and may involve optimizing hormones, nutrition, and vitamin levels as well as an evaluation by a dermatologist who specializes in hair loss.

Osteoporosis

Osteoporosis is a progressive thinning of bones that occurs silently and painlessly until a bone breaks. Osteoporosis affects about forty-four million American men and women, accounting for 55 percent of the population age 50 and older. One of every two women will suffer from osteoporosis. Risk factors for osteoporosis are

- ❖ Age and female sex
- ❖ Family history
- ❖ White or Asian ethnic background
- ❖ Small body frame
- ❖ History of amenorrhea (no periods for over six months)
- ❖ Anorexia or history of anorexia
- ❖ History of steroid use

❖ Smoking and excessive alcohol

❖ Limited calcium and Vitamin D intake.

Building up bone density prior to menopause is the best strategy for preventing osteoporosis. Once menopause occurs, hormone replacement has been shown to help prevent breakage and strengthen bones (NIH, 2007).

Cardiovascular Disease (CVD)

Heart disease is the number one cause of death for American women. Estrogen is a powerful cholesterol-reducing drug. It can help increase your good cholesterol (HDL) and decrease your bad cholesterol (LDL). As women enter menopause, decreasing estrogen levels worsen women's cholesterol and increase their risk for heart disease. By age 65, the percentage of women dying from CVD is greater than the number of men who die from CVD.

HORMONE REPLACEMENT THERAPY FOR WOMEN

Many problems associated with menopause can be prevented and improved with hormone replacement therapy (HRT). However, not all women are candidates. The types of hormones used as well as the age at which a woman starts hormone replacement are important.

Hormone replacement is controversial due to the findings of the Women's Health Initiative (WHI). This was a randomized, controlled trial of 161,809 women between the ages of 50 and 79. All of these women, regardless of their medical conditions, were given the same dose of synthetic hormones: Premarin and Provera. The trial was stopped prematurely because of increases in cardiovascular disease, breast cancer, and all-cause mortality (Rousseau, 2002).

Because of this finding, many doctors stopped prescribing hormone therapies. Since then, many researchers have reviewed the findings and disagreed with the results while agreeing that the WHI study had many flaws. The average age of women entering the study was 63.3 years, ten years past the beginning of menopause when true risk reduction can occur. Furthermore, only 10 percent of the participants were 50 to 54 years old; only 16 percent were less than five years after the onset of menopause. Many of the women had medical conditions that would make them poor candidates for hormone replacement. In the WHI study, 36 percent had hypertension, 49 percent were current or past smokers, and 34 percent had a BMI greater than 30. For years, doctors have used these factors as standard contraindications for hormonal contraceptives. To summarize, the women in the WHI study were older, postmeno-pausal women who had significantly increased risk factors for cardiovascular disease (Cobin, 2006).

Another commonly-referred-to clinical trial is the heart disease and hormone re-placement study called the Heart and Estrogen/Progestin Replacement Study (HERS) and the Nurses' Study; it found that HRT did not work as a secondary prevention tool for cardiovascular events (Hulley, 1998). (Secondary prevention describes using medi-cations or treatments in patients with chronic disease to prevent that disease process from worsening.) This trial highlights that for women who ALREADY have heart dis-ease, hormone replacement is not helpful.

Since these trials, researchers have studied the benefits of hormone replacement. The most recent consensus statement came at the Zurich Summit of 2008 for meno-pause, where forty of the world's leading menopause experts reviewed public percep-tions, risks, and benefits. They concluded:

Cardiovascular issues: Combined estrogen and progesterone do not increase chronic heart disease risk in healthy women aged 50-59; estrogen alone actually de-creases the risk for this group.

Breast cancer: Certain types of HRT (combined estrogen and progesterone) can lead to a slightly increased risk of breast cancer. However, this is minimal in relation to other breast cancer risk factors. Women with no prior use of estrogen alone actu-ally had no increased risk for breast cancer in the WHI. Short-to-medium term use of estrogen-only HRT does not show this effect. Each woman should discuss her general health and risk factors (such as family history, smoking, etc.) with her doctor, but gen-erally, healthy women (e.g., with no other breast cancer risk factors) entering meno-pause should have no fears of breast cancer due to HRT.

Bone Health: HRT is effective in maintaining bone health in 50 to 59-year-old post-menopausal women.

Cognition: HRT does not impair cognition in healthy women aged 50-59 and may even delay decreases in cognitive functioning in this group (International Menopause Society, 2008).

Thus, for healthy women, I strongly support the use of hormone replacement to help with controlling hot flashes and mood swings, improving focus, concentration, energy, and vitality, reducing the risk of heart disease and of osteoporosis, maintain-ing weight and tone, and having a more youthful look!

What Type of Hormones Should You Take?

Once again, this is controversial. The WHI Study, Nurse's Study, and HERS study used synthetic hormones, which the body views as foreign. They may not enter the same metabolic pathway as bio-identical hormones. Biologically identical hormones are derived from plants, such as the wild yam or soybean plant. Wild yams and soybeans are rich in precursor molecules that can be converted into progesterone and estrogen whose molecular structures are the same as those produced naturally in the human body.

The following lists contraindications to hormone replacement, but speak with your Age Management physician to see if you are a candidate.

Relative Contraindications to Estrogen Therapy Include:
- ❖ Family history of breast cancer (outside immediate family)
- ❖ Benign breast disease
- ❖ Past history of recurrent thromboembolisms (blood clots)
- ❖ Moderate or severe endometriosis
- ❖ Enlarging fibroids or fibroids that produce heavy bleeding

Absolute Contraindications to Estrogen Therapy Include:
- ❖ Presence of non-eradicated endometrial cancer
- ❖ History of breast cancer
- ❖ Cancer history in first-degree relatives
- ❖ Active thrombosis (blood clot)
- ❖ Acute liver disease or chronic liver failure
- ❖ Unexplained vaginal bleeding
- ❖ Being pregnant

Contraindications to Progesterone Therapy Include:
- ❖ Allergy to progesterone, progesterone-like drugs, or inactive ingredients
- ❖ Past or present blood clots
- ❖ Liver disease
- ❖ Known or suspected cancer of the breast or reproductive organs
- ❖ Unusual bleeding from the vagina, not evaluated by a physician
- ❖ Miscarriage with suspected tissue remaining in the uterus
- ❖ Currently breastfeeding

TESTOSTERONE FOR WOMEN

Just as testosterone is important for men's health, testosterone is critical for women's health. Women produce testosterone mostly in the ovaries and a small amount in the adrenal glands. Women with adrenal failure or surgical removal of their ovaries suffer from low testosterone levels, which the medical community has agreed is an indication for testosterone (Miller, 2006). However, for menopausal women, the general medical community is still arguing whether or not testosterone is needed. Emerging evidence demonstrates that women can benefit from testosterone therapy in terms of sexual health, libido, muscle mass, bone mass, and cognitive functions.

Testosterone therapy is an off-label treatment for women. Off-label treatments are common in medicine; they occur when physicians use a medication for a reason outside the one indicated by the FDA. For example, physicians use seizure medications to prevent migraines. Physicians use testosterone as an off-label treatment for the common symptoms that occur with menopause.

The most common reason that I use testosterone is to increase a woman's sexual libido and interest. The sexual health of my patients is an important part of health and mental well-being and a key component in maintaining intimate relationships. Clinical trials involving postmenopausal women who have libido loss have demonstrated that adding testosterone to estrogen significantly improved sexual functioning, including libido, sexual desire, and arousal, as well as sexual frequency and satisfaction. In controlled clinical trials of up to two years, women receiving testosterone therapy tolerated it well and had no serious side effects (Bolour, 2005).

Other possible benefits of testosterone are that it can help build bone and muscle mass and help reduce body fat. These are important concerns in women's health. Low testosterone levels have been correlated with an increase in osteoporosis. No studies evaluate just testosterone and osteoporosis, but the studies that have evaluated testosterone and estrogen together have shown an increase or a comparable change in bone density (Pompei, 2006). The "normal aging" process causes lean muscle to be replaced with fat. While exercise can slow this down, most women (as men) eventually hit a plateau. If unabated, women begin to lose muscle mass. Remember, women have one-tenth the testosterone that men do, so a small reduction in muscle mass due to lower testosterone and the effects of aging can have serious consequences on overall health. And as she loses muscle with aging and then with hormone loss, a woman's body fat will increase, which will then increase her risk of heart disease. This loss of muscle also accelerates bone loss, which increases her risk of osteoporosis further. As stated earlier, one out of two women suffers from osteoporosis, so preventative actions are important (NIH, 2007).

How does testosterone affect a woman's risk of heart disease? Recent studies have shown that transdermal testosterone (i.e., given in a patch or cream) does not affect her cholesterol profile. Oral testosterone has been shown to decrease HDL (good testosterone) for women (Miller K. , 2001).

Careful consultation with an Age Management physician or a physician who understands hormone replacement therapy, its side effects, and its monitoring is an important aspect of evaluating your hormones. As with all medications, testosterone therapy has risks. Contraindications to testosterone therapy are pregnancy (or even considering pregnancy), breastfeeding, testosterone-secreting tumors and hyperandrogenemia (i.e., women with high levels of testosterone), breast cancer, uterine cancer, liver disease, and cardiovascular disease (Miller K. , 2001; NAMS, 2005). A recent review of the Nurses' Health Study also showed that there may be an increased risk for breast cancer in women with testosterone and estrogen therapy. Please remember, though, that this study used synthetic hormones rather than bio-identical ones. Further studies are needed, but it is important to discuss with your physician your risk for breast cancer when considering hormone replacement (Tamimi, 2006).

DIHYDROEPIANDOSTERONE (DHEA)

Made in our adrenal glands, DHEA is one of the building blocks needed for testosterone in men and women. DHEA is a critical hormone to help slow aging. DHEA levels are the same in women and men until about age 50. Then men have a gradual decline in men and women a steeper drop-off (K. Miller, 2001). DHEA production is maximal between 20 and 30 years of age, and then begins to decline by 2 percent per year. By age 80, we have only 20 percent of the DHEA that we had in our 20s (K. Miller , 2001).

Epidemiological data indicate an inverse relationship between serum DHEA and the frequency of cancer, Alzheimer's disease, cardiovascular disease (in men only), other age-related disorders, immune function, and the progression of HIV infection (Pepping, 2000). Emerging studies indicate that DHEA may improve immune function by helping increase the number of cells that fight off cancer cells. More studies are needed to show the true relationship between DHEA and cancer. But for now, it seems there may be a positive correlation.

DHEA supplementation has been used in patients with low serum DHEA levels, chronic disease, adrenal exhaustion, and systemic lupus erythematosus (SLE), as well as those on steroid therapy. It has improved bone density in postmenopausal women, symptoms of depression, and depressed mood and fatigue in HIV patients (Pepping, 2000).

Recently, a study was conducted on men and women aged 45 to 65 years who had depression beginning in mid-life. The depression of people who used DHEA improved, and the authors concluded that DHEA may be an effective treatment for mid-life depression (Schmidt, 2005).

The *European Journal of Endocrinology* reported definite short-term benefits of DHEA, such as improvements in mood, well-being, and sexual dysfunction (more with women than with men) (Gurnell, 2001). And the *American Endocrinologist* reported bone mass density increases in older men and women who used DHEA for one year (Jankowski, 2006).

As with other hormones, DHEA is currently being studied for its effects on aging. For now, I recommend DHEA if people are symptomatic and have low levels. Since it can be bought over the counter, it is important to use pharmaceutical grade DHEA to achieve optimal results and minimize side effects. Check your levels before and after therapy to confirm that you are at optimal levels. Contraindications to DHEA are hormone-sensitive cancers of the prostate, uterus, and breast as well as a history of deep venous blood clots. Once again, please check with your Age Management Specialist or doctor, since using DHEA is controversial.

THYROID HORMONE

The thyroid is one of the most common hormones physicians check because it causes vague symptoms of fatigue and depression. An underactive thyroid causes low energy and fatigue (especially in the morning), difficulty losing weight, cold feet and hands, depression, constipation, dry skin, menstrual abnormalities, infertility, palpitations, shortness of breath, dry skin, hair loss, and slowed cognitive functions. Even with all these symptoms, it is still one of the most underdiagnosed conditions in adults.

The thyroid gland is responsible for your metabolism rate. When thyroid levels are low, replacing thyroid hormones can help patients feel better and more energetic and help with depression, weight maintenance, and menses regulation.

The most common test physicians use to diagnose thyroid conditions is the thyroid stimulating hormone (TSH). This is the signal the brain sends to the thyroid gland to produce two hormones (called T4 [thyroxine] or T3]triiodothyronine]) that work on the rest of the body. Your body converts T4 to T3, but when you are stressed or get older, this conversion does not always occur (Becker, 2001).

A traditional physician usually does not check your full thyroid profile because it is not "cost effective." However, emerging data shows that the full panel is the best way to evaluate the thyroid. It is important to check all thyroid functions because low levels of T3 and free T3 are independent predictors of mortality in the general population (Iervasi, 2003). T3 plays a strong role in controlling the cardiovascular system and peripheral arteries as well as in kidney disease (Iervasi, 2003; Carrero, 2007). Emerging science is beginning to show that low levels of T3 are an important marker of poor health (Iervasi, 2007).

Even with emerging evidence of the benefits of treating low thyroid levels, it is controversial in traditional medicine to treat subclinical thyroid disorders (Surks, 2004). (Subclinical indicates a borderline level of disease in which people may or may not have symptoms.) As an Age Management physician, I recommend treating subclinical hypothyroid states and low T3 syndromes because they have been associated with poor health and an increased risk of heart disease.

However, too much thyroid medication can increase your risk of hyperthyroidism, which can thin bones and increase your risk of arrhythmias and heart dysfunction (Wilson, 2005). As with everything we have discussed, we are always striving for the balance and optimization of health. We are not aiming for extremes of health, but its optimization. This occurs with physicians who are experienced with Optimal Health and have the time and desire to educate their patients about risks and benefits.

Check with your Age Management Specialist or doctor, since treatment is controversial.

HUMAN GROWTH HORMONE

Human growth hormone is the master hormone that affects all other hormones, organs, and cells in our bodies. It has amazing reparative and restorative powers that can reverse cellular and tissue damage as well as help rejuvenate failing organs. Growth hormone (GH) is responsible for growth and healing, immune function, increasing muscle mass and strength, minimizing body fat, controlling cholesterol, increasing bone strength, and helping us maintain high energy levels, including sexual energy and performance.

Growth hormone secretion is affected by many factors such as exercise, stress, emotional excitement, diet, and aging (Becker, 2001). After puberty, growth hormone levels begin to fall at the rate of 15 percent per decade for reasons that are poorly understood (Becker, 2001). By age 60, most of us produce only 25 percent of the growth hormone we produced at age 21. This age-related decline in growth hormone produces many undesirable changes, including increased body fat, a loss of bone and muscle tissue and strength, declines in cardiac function and exercise performance, declines in mood and a sense of well-being, and poor wound healing.

Age alone is not the only cause of declining growth hormone levels. Excess body fat also lowers growth hormone levels, creating a vicious cycle of increased abdominal fat which further drives down growth hormone levels (Vahl, 1996). As discussed earlier, increased abdominal fat is associated with an increased risk of insulin resistance, diabetes, high cholesterol, heart disease, heart attacks, and strokes.

The signs and symptoms of GH declines are the same as aging. There is an increase in body fat (especially around the trunk), a decrease in muscular strength, a decrease in bone density, and a decrease in energy and vitality. There is a decrease in psychosocial well-being, depression, anxiety, and social isolation as well as drier skin, an increase in wrinkles, and decreases in sweating and body temperature regulation (Becker, 2001).

Improving growth hormone levels can dramatically slow, prevent, or even reverse all this by working to repair, heal, and rejuvenate at the cellular level. Dramatic improvements in muscle mass, bone strength, exercise endurance, brain function, and the integrity of hair, nails, and skin will occur with increased growth hormone levels. Additional benefits include a resolution of depression, an increased quality of sleep, a sense of well-being, initiative, and an improved libido and sex life, as well as greater overall mental and physical health. Growth hormone supplementation can improve cholesterol levels, which decreases the risk of cardiovascular disease (Molitich, 2006). Growth hormone can also improve immunity which scientists believe can prevent cancer and increase longevity.

Growth hormone supplementation is controversial. At this time, it is indicated only for adults who have a deficiency in growth hormone. If your growth hormone levels do not fall into this low range and you do not have symptoms of growth hormone deficiency, GH supplementation is not an option for you.

In my holistic practice, patients who follow the Optimal Health Program can increase their growth hormone levels naturally by just living better. This occurs slowly over a year's time, using each spoke of the Personal Wellness Wheel™. My patients feel significantly better without ever using growth hormone. Their levels will never be the same as those using growth hormone, but they are high enough to improve health and their quality of life. Growth hormone release is naturally affected by the spokes in your Personal Wellness Wheel™ such as exercise, nutrition, reducing stress, deep sleep, and decreasing your body fat. As you optimize these elements of the Personal Wellness Wheel™, you, like many of my patients, may improve your growth hormone levels. Below are the mechanisms for how this happens.

NATURAL METHODS OF INCREASING YOUR HUMAN GROWTH HORMONE

Exercising

Exercising can improve growth hormone levels. Acute increases in growth hormone levels occur with heavy resistance training and with intense running and cycling (Hornum, 1997). But most people usually do not exercise, and if they do, they do not perform workouts intense enough to release growth hormone. The first step is to improve your exercise capacity and strength. Engage in more strenuous workouts as you optimize your exercise routine. You can use the charts provided in Chapter Four, visit us online at www.optimalhealthtoday.com for training tips, and/or work with a qualified personal trainer. Walking is a great first step, but to actually release more growth hormone and reach Optimal Health, you need to do more.

While growth hormone is naturally released during and after exercise, it is sensitive to increases in sugar. I recommend drinking water (not sports drinks, which have hidden sugars) and waiting one to two hours after exercising to eat, thereby optimizing the full release of growth hormone. Thirty to sixty minutes before exercising, eat a protein-dense meal to prevent fatigue. This is contrary to what most of us have heard, but in this Optimal Health Program, we are integrating the latest knowledge of hormones and exercise to slow the aging process.

Good Nutrition

With the aging process, growth hormone levels decrease, resulting in increased fat deposits, especially in the midsection, which worsens insulin resistance. Remember, insulin signals your body to move glucose from the blood into the organs where it is used as energy. When you have insulin resistance, your body no longer responds to insulin, and your insulin and glucose levels begin to rise. These increased levels set up a vicious cycle in which the elevated insulin and glucose levels increase body weight and fat, which then further drives down growth hormone. Eating a low glycemic diet like the Mediterranean Diet can help keep insulin and glucose levels low so that they do not affect growth hormone levels.

Decreasing Stress

Growth hormone levels decrease with stress. Stress causes the release of cortisol, which stops or slows the release of growth hormone. To deal with stress, read Chapter Seven on mindfulness and make meditation a part of your life. Do yoga which is meditation in motion. Yoga's focus on breathing and quieting the body can reduce cortisol levels and improve overall health. I also recommend practicing generosity and compassion on a regular basis. The act of giving can make people feel better and reduce their stress.

Getting Enough Deep Sleep

Growth hormone is released at night, while we are in deep sleep. If you cannot get deep sleep, your growth hormone will not be released. If this is occasional, it is okay, but if falling asleep or staying asleep is a concern, please speak with your physician since this is affecting your health.

Decreasing Body Fat

As you follow the Optimal Health Program, you will have less body fat, which stops that vicious cycle of falling growth hormone levels. You lose body fat through exercising, eating better, managing your stress, and improving your sleep.

NATURAL WAYS TO BOOST YOUR HUMAN GROWTH HORMONE

- ❖ Get eight hours of deep sleep per night. Human growth hormone production relies on a good night's rest.
- ❖ Drink as little alcohol (a high glycemic food) as possible.
- ❖ Eat organic protein (such as chicken, fish, turkey, lentils, blackeyed peas, or soybeans) with every meal. The amino acid lysine in protein stimulates the production of human growth hormone.
- ❖ Eat more fruits and veggies; eat two servings per day of multigrains.
- ❖ Avoid anything that contains sugar.
- ❖ Engage in regular exercise, including yoga.
- ❖ Keep stress to a minimum, as it uses up your human growth hormone.
- ❖ Be grateful and give to others.
- ❖ Lower your exposure to pollution and pesticides, which can affect your endocrine system.

BUILDING SPOKE FIVE
OF YOUR PERSONAL WELLNESS WHEEL™

☐ Educate yourself: Carefully review the information in this chapter and realize that making a choice for hormone replacement is contingent on many health factors and must be discussed with your Age Management Specialist or your personal physician. HRT has many benefits and is effective in appropriately selected patients. Also review the literature we have presented in the appendix at the end of this workbook.

☐ Make a list of your symptoms using the chart below. If you answer yes to more than seven, you should consider having your hormone levels checked.

Symptom	Yes	No
Feeling tired		
Loss of energy		
Feeling depressed		
Feeling moody		
Weight increases		
Difficulty losing weight		
Difficulty improving muscle mass		
Do you have osteopenia or osteoporosis?		
Loss of libido		
Difficulty focusing		
Difficulty concentrating		
Difficulty with memory		
Getting sick often		
Do you have diabetes?		
Do you have liver disease?		
Do you have lupus/rheumatoid arthritis or a collagen vascular disease?		
Do you have heart disease?		
For men: Do you have morning erections?		
For men: Do you have erectile dysfunction?		
For women: Do you have hot flashes?		
For women: Do you have vaginal dryness?		

❑ Consider asking your physician to order the following blood work for you and record the results:

Labs to have checked:

Laboratory Test	Men	Women
Thyroid stimulating hormone		
Free T4		
Free T3		
DHEA		
Insulin Growth Factor 1		
Cortisol		
Total Testosterone		
Free Testosterone		
PSA (men only)		
Luteinizing hormone		
Follicle stimulating hormone (women only)		
Insulin		
Progesterone (women only)		
Estradiol		
Dihydrotestosterone (men only)		

❖ A caution with lab testing: Your insurance company may not cover all of the laboratory tests in the above table since they are for Optimal Health rather than the commonly performed basic lab panels. This laboratory testing can be expensive, and you may be responsible for any out-of-pocket costs. It is important to ask your physician what lab tests will not be covered to avoid any financial surprise.

❖ Also, what is considered a normal level will vary from facility to facility. It is best to speak with a healthcare professional who specializes in hormone replacement to see what your laboratory information means.

❑ Remember, controversy surrounds HRT, and the information presented here is for your education only; you must consult with a qualified medical professional to help you make your decision.

Beauty is Eternity gazing at itself in the mirror.

~ Khalil Gibran

YOUR AGELESS SKIN: IMPROVING YOUR SKIN AT ANY AGE

In Eastern philosophy, we look for balance between internal health, for example, how well we feel, and external health, meaning how we look. In our society today, we recognize that appearance influences our self-image and the way we are perceived by others.

Skin is the largest visible organ of our bodies and a visual history of how well we have taken care of ourselves and how healthy we are. Inflammation in our bodies can manifest in our skin as acne, rosacea, uneven skin tones, wrinkles, or other common medical skin conditions. The goal of this chapter is to help you understand how to have the best skin at whatever age you are.

How we look is an important part of the Personal Wellness Wheel™ because when we feel good about ourselves, we are more likely to engage in the healthy behaviors that create Optimal Health. Every day I see patients begin to improve their health as they feel more confident about their appearance. This is not vanity, but the desire in all of us to look good and feel great. Good, healthy skin is part of that.

In this chapter, you will learn the following:

○ Structure of the Skin
○ Intrinsic Skin Aging
○ Extrinsic Skin Aging
○ Effects of Aging
○ Skin Care Products
○ Advanced Skin Care Treatments
○ Common Skin Conditions
○ Finding Your Skin Care Specialist
○ Hair Removal

STRUCTURE OF THE SKIN

The skin has three different layers:

1. Epidermis: the top layer of skin. It is regenerated every six to eight weeks. New cells from the bottom of this layer migrate up; the old cells, which are now dead, are sloughed off by the skin.
2. Dermis: the middle part of the skin. Collagen and elastin fibers are produced here to help maintain the skin's strength and flexibility.
3. Hypodermis: The subcutis is the deepest layer of the skin, consisting of a network of collagen and fat cells that help conserve your body's heat and protect your body from injury by acting as a "shock absorber."

INTRINSIC SKIN AGING

Aging of the skin is a complex phenomena that involves both intrinsic and extrinsic changes influences on the skin.

Intrinsic skin aging is the normal wear and tear *within* our skin that our bodies experience. We lose collagen and elastin at the rate of 1 percent every year after the age of 24. As we age, intrinsic skin aging results in fine lines, dryer appearing skin, paler or uneven skin tones, skin laxity, and benign skin lesions.

EXTRINSIC SKIN AGING

Extrinsic skin aging results from influences outside the skin, such as sun exposure, tanning, smoking, and hormonal loss. A cumulative process that occurs in addition to intrinsic skin changes due to aging, it results in more damage. As men age and experience andropause (male menopause), their skin gradually changes. Because menopause creates a more sudden shift in hormones, women's skin can age faster because collagen and elastin rapidly break down. The results are fine to deep lines, discoloration, sallowness, dry texture, tone loss, dyspigmentation, sagging, leathery-appearing skin, and an increased chance of skin cancer.

EFFECTS OF AGING

Aging affects each layer of the skin differently. As we age, each layer of our skin gradually atrophies. The epidermis thins, and the natural shedding or exfoliation of this top layer of skin slows each decade, leaving the skin appearing uneven, dryer, and duller. The dermis produces less collagen and elastin. With photoaging, damage from UV sunrays causes abnormal tissue to accumulate. This diminishes collagen and further weakens and thins it, leading to both fine and deep wrinkles as well as the leathery appearance seen in sun-exposed areas. As the other skin layers thin and atrophy, gravity begins to affect the hypodermis and slowly pulls the subcutaneous fat down.

For instance, as we age, our facial structure changes. In our 20s and 30s, the fullest part of our face is our cheeks, and our jawline is naturally tight, forming an inverted triangle. In our 40s and 50s, as the aging process begins, the dermis thins and atrophies. The pull of gravity and the breakdown of the dermis causes the fat in the cheeks to travel slowly down to the jawline. We begin to have a more square or rectangular shaped face and thinner lips as a result. As fat begins to accumulate, we can have unevenness in the jawline. As we approach our 60s, the fat is now at the jawline, causing more of the jowling, turkey-neck appearance and sagging. The end result is that we have an upright triangle rather than the inverted triangle we started with as a young person.

Now that you understand the skin changes that occur with age, how can you slow them? Most importantly, stay out of the sun and tanning booths! Most of the damage done by the sun and tanning occurs before we are 18 years of age—when most of us don't listen to anyone! But stopping photoaging at any age will help. The next step is not to smoke or pick at your skin. Finally, reduce your alcohol consumption!

Lifestyle changes are vitally important to the health of your skin. Take better care of yourself, and your health will be reflected in better skin.

SKIN CARE PRODUCTS

To slow the aging process, start early. Fixing changes that have already occurred is much more expensive than preventing them in the first place. The choice of skin care products is one of the most important decisions that you can make to help slow the aging process.

The dermatological products that work are the ones that have been proven over time. Spend your money on pharmaceutical or physician grade products; they are stronger and penetrate deeper.

To discuss which products are best for you, meet with a skin care specialist who can explain the best products for you and how to use them. The following are the products I use and have seen the best results with.

Vitamin C serum is the most important topical treatment that you need to PREVENT a wrinkle. The Vitamin C serum must be in the right alpha-tocopheral shape, in a serum form, and at the right pH to work. Ask your skin care expert to recommend a good Vitamin C product.

Alpha hydroxy acid (AHA) helps the skin exfoliate because as we age, the natural exfoliation process slows down, leaving the skin dull and sallow. A daily AHA product will keep your skin exfoliated and healthier.

Hydroquinone is for dark pigmentation. Hydroquinone stops melanocytes from being overactive and scarring the skin and helps even your skin tone. I do not recommend that people use anything stronger than 4 percent (the prescription grade level) unless advised by your skin care expert. Do not use hydroquinone during pregnancy.

Other products that can help lighten your skin are vitamin C, kojic acid, and licorice, but these are significantly weaker than hydroquinone.

Retin-A or retinoic acids help the skin exfoliate. Over time, it also helps reduce discoloration, especially when it works with hydroquinone. Furthermore, Retin-A 0.1% cream (the highest strength) can actually correct a skin cell's damaged DNA if used consistently for more than one year; this can decrease your risk of skin cancer in the areas to which it is applied.

Using Retin-A (generic: tretinoin) is a lifelong commitment, so start slowly and let your skin build up its tolerance. You will need to consult with your skin care specialist to find the best form of retinoic acid for you. Remember to start with a mild form; as your skin becomes stronger, move to the next level so you can optimize your results. The goal is to use this on a regular basis to improve your skin, as short-term use does not change the skin.

Broad-spectrum sunblock is an important skin care product. Broad-spectrum sunblock protects you against both UVA and UVB rays. UVB rays are much weaker than UVA and cannot penetrate through glass. For these, SPF provides your protection. UVA rays are much stronger. They can penetrate through glass and are also given off by the fluorescent lighting found in many buildings; you are not protected just because you are indoors. The protection you need against UVA is a physical barrier such as zinc or titanium. SPF alone is not sufficient. Ask your pharmacist or skin care specialist which sunblocks are best for you.

ADVANCED SKIN CARE TREATMENTS

Advanced skin care treatments have rapidly flooded the market. They are the fastest growing part of the cosmetic surgery and medical boom. The treatments you can use will vary depending on your skin tone and skin condition. You must speak with a qualified skin care specialist to learn what is best for you.

Today, there are many options for skin care. You can go to a day spa, medical spa, dermatology office, cosmetic medicine office, plastic surgeon, or maybe your primary care physician or gynecologist. Day spas in general do not offer medical-grade treatments because no physician is involved. Medical grade treatments must have physician involvement; how much involvement varies. And remember this: The treatment is only as good as the technician doing it. Many places do not provide extensive training. You should check the staff credentials and training at any facility where you intend to receive advanced skin care consultation or treatment.

To understand advanced skin care, you need to understand what your problem is and how long you have had it. For example, long-term, deep sun damage will require a stronger treatment. The most important thing you can do is educate yourself about your skin condition and its available treatments. Feel comfortable asking about training and experience. Most importantly, make sure you feel that the staff listens to your concerns and explains what you can expect. If they promise too much, it's probably too good to be true. Advanced skin care treatments help improve skin, but there is no such thing as a miracle in the realm of non-surgical procedures.

TREATMENTS

Chemical Peel

Chemical peels can treat fine lines and wrinkles as well as improve acne and other brown spots that might have occurred with time and sun exposure. Chemical peels can brighten and even your skin as well as improve its overall tone.

There are four types of chemical peels.

❑ Topical peel: This is what you can buy in stores without seeing a specialist. They have not been shown to be clinically effective.

❑ Superficial Progressive Peel: This penetrates into the first layer and the top of the second layer of skin. Peels have different strengths, so as you increase your strength, you can get a deeper peel that will enhance your skin. Superficial peels DO NOT have any down time. You may return to work that day.

❑ Medium Depth Peel: This penetrates into the second layer of skin, requiring some anesthesia for comfort and three to seven days of down time. This is for people who have more extensive sun damage and wrinkles.

❑ Deep Peel: This penetrates deep into the dermis, the second layer of skin. It is used for people suffering from actinic keratoses (precancer lesions) and severe scarring. It requires sedation and a considerable recovery time.

Microdermabrasion

Microdermabrasion is a mechanical exfoliation of the skin to stimulate the growth of healthier skin. People who benefit from microdermabrasion are people with

❖ Blotchy and uneven skin

❖ Hyperpigmented acne scars and/or other scars

❖ Blackheads and whiteheads

❖ Fine lines

❖ Oily skin

❖ Those who want overall more healthy and clear skin.

Lasers

In general, lasers penetrate more deeply than the treatments above (except for the deep peels). There are two types: ablative and non-ablative lasers.

❑ <u>Non-ablative lasers</u> are an intense pulse light treatment. **Skin rejuvenation lasers** or photofacial treatments are non-ablative laser treatments. They are popular because they involve no downtime. They bypass the surface of the skin (the epidermis) and treat the layer underneath (the first part of the dermis) with heat. The skin responds as if it was repairing a wound; it regenerates new skin with no damage to the outermost layer of skin. These lasers help stimulate new collagen and elastin and decrease visible superficial blood vessels. For optimal results, they require multiple sessions. I like using them on lighter skin tones and clients who suffer from rosacea. If you have a darker skin tone and wish to use these treatments, first ask if the facility's laser can be used on your skin type; if yes, pre-treat the skin with hydroquinone and Retin-A for six weeks.

❑ <u>Ablative lasers</u>:

■ These are **Erbium:Yag** or **CO2** lasers that penetrate deeply into the dermis to build new collagen and elastin.

■ **Fractional laser skin treatments** represent a new science and category of cosmetic skin surgery, offering clients the positive results of ablative resurfacing with the low-impact benefits of non-ablative therapies. Unlike old ablative lasers that removed the top layer of skin, fractional laser treatments produce tiny, microscopic sites of thermal impact separated by areas of unaffected, healthy tissue. The spared healthy tissue between treatment zones contains viable cells that promote rapid healing of the outer skin layers. At the same time, the treated area penetrates deeply into the skin to help build and remodel collagen. They involve a few days of down time during which you will look sunburned, followed by another week of peeling and flaking.

   Many laser companies state that darker complexions should not use this laser; however at our Institute, we have experience with darker skin tones and use this fractional technology well. If you have a darker skin tone, please make sure your physician has experience with your skin type.

■ **Skin tightening lasers**: Skin begins to sag because of collagen and elastin loss. The jury is still out on the overall results of skin tightening lasers. If you have a lot of sagging or redundancy, the best treatment is surgery. But if the problem is just starting, these lasers can be beneficial for prevention and maintenance. The best approach to sagging skin is combining laser treatments that

help build collagen and elastin and at the same time tighten the skin.
■ **Body shaping/cellulite**: This is the newest field in the aesthetic market. These treatments work by removing small, unwanted fat cells, trying to dissolve the fat using chemicals, and/or reducing the size of fat cells. All these treatments can improve the bodies of people in their right body mass index, but they are not miracle treatments. They may help you improve your body, but will not give you a new body! As with all treatments, combining these treatments provides the best results, and it takes about four to six treatments to achieve good results.

Injectable Therapies

To understand which type of injectable therapy is best for you, talk with your physician.

Product Name	Used For	How it Works	Lasts For	Side Effects
Botox®	Lines in motion on/ around the forehead, eyes, lips, Marionette lines, & turkey neck	Weakens and paralyzes the muscle	3-6 months	Bruising, redness, headache, flu-like symptoms, numbness at injection site
Hyaluronic Fillers: Juvederm™ Restylane® Perlane® Captique™ Hylaform	Mild to moderate creases around the mouth, hollow under eyes, lips	Hyaluronic-based soft tissue fillers used to increase volume/ fullness	Juvederm™ 9-12 months; the rest 4-6 months	Bruising, redness, swelling, can be visible if injected too close to skin
Collagen Fillers: Evolence® (new) Artefill® Cosmoplast® Cosmoderm®	For smile lines and other facial lines	Collagen-based so can restore volume and replace declining collagen	Evolence® 6-12 months; Artefill® permanent; Others 3-4 months	Bruising, swelling, redness

Radiesse®	For smile lines and volume replacement; not for lips	Calcium-based, water-based gel that stimulates collagen production and serves as filler	About 1 year	Bruising, swelling, redness, discomfort at injection site
Sculptra™	For replacing facial volume lost with age and HIV wasting	Made of poly L Lactic acid to build collagen and add volume	About 2 years	Bruising, swelling, redness
Fat Injections	To add facial volume, to fill lines and enhance lips	Taking fat from one body part (e.g., abdomen) and re-injecting it in another area	Can be 3-6 months, longer, or permanent	Bruising, swelling, redness

COMMON SKIN CONDITIONS

RED SKIN

This refers to clients that have rosacea, vasculitis, or strong red undertones. Their skin often has broken capillaries, small spider veins (telangiectasia), rhinophyma (thickened skin on the nose), red papules/pustules, or easy flushing.

Treatment Options
- ❏ Laser skin rejuvenation is the best treatment. A fractional laser treatment is good after a skin rejuvenation treatment to help build up skin thickness. For severe rosacea, topical antibiotic treatments and oral antibiotics can help, but recent literature reports that laser treatments can provide better results than long-term antibiotic use.
- ❏ Chemical peels can help even skin tones and texture.
- ❏ Laser: For broken capillaries, a laser vein treatment can be very helpful.

Brown Spots/Discoloration

This refers to the following:

❖ <u>Sun spots</u>: Liver or age spots (called lentigos) frequently occur on the face, neck, upper chest, and arms.

  ❖ <u>Post inflammatory hyperpigmentation/discoloration</u>: A common occurrence that may result from a skin injury, such as acne, rashes, or generalized skin trauma.

❖ <u>Freckles</u>: The body's natural response to sun exposure, freckles will often fade after sun exposure is diminished or eliminated.

❖ <u>Melasma</u>: Darkening of the skin often caused by hormonal changes such as those with pregnancy, menopause, irregular periods, or hormonal contraception.

❖ <u>Acne</u>: Scarring can result from acne.

Treatment Options

❑ If mild, use microdermabrasion or peels.

❑ If mild to moderate and on lighter skin types, use skin rejuvenation laser.

❑ If mild to moderate with darker skin types, pretreat with Retin-A and hydroquinone for six weeks. Then use fractional laser or some skin rejuvenation lasers.

❑ If moderate to severe, a fractional laser can be used as well as medium and deep peels. Treatment should be discussed with your skin care specialist. If you have darker skin, I recommend using hydroquinone and Retin-A for six weeks and working with someone who is comfortable with your complexion.

Acneic Skin

Acne occurs when oil-secreting glands become blocked and inflamed. Acne can occur on the face, neck, shoulders, chest, back, and even the thighs.

There are many different types of acne:

❖ <u>Whiteheads</u> are infected hair follicles that are still closed on the top of the skin.

❖ <u>Blackheads</u> are infected hair follicles that are open to the air. The black color comes not from dirt, but from air exposure.

❖ <u>Pustules (pimples)</u> are inflamed areas that contain pus and have a red base.

❖ <u>Papules</u> are small red bumps that do not contain pus.

❖ <u>Cysts</u> are pustules that grow larger and deeper, which may cause scarring.

❖ <u>Nodules</u> are large, painful deep lesions within the skin.

The exact cause of acne is not known, but doctors believe that it is caused by several factors.

❖ Hormone levels: Androgens (male hormone levels) found in both men and women can cause acne. Acne may be due to high levels of these hormones or because of an age-related fluctuation such as puberty or menopause.

❖ Changing hormone levels: Acne outbreaks or new acne can be seen in pregnant women and women who suddenly stop or start a birth control method.

❖ Family history of acne: If one or both of your parents had acne, the probability that you will suffer from acne increases.

❖ Friction/Pressure: Anything that can put pressure on an affected area such as cell phones, backpacks, helmets, purses, hats, and/or clothing can cause acne.

❖ Picking or scrubbing the skin too hard can worsen acne.

❖ Environmental factors that increase pollution or humidity can make acne worse.

❖ Diet: Once dismissed as folklore by physicians, there is emerging evidence that your diet may contribute to acne. Various studies are now evaluating high gly-cemic and fat diets and diets high in dairy as causes of acne.

Severity of Acne and Treatment Options

❖ Mild acne describes skin with a few whiteheads, blackheads, and/or pustules. Mild acne can be controlled using a good home-care regimen and occasional peels to improve the penetration of products.

❖ Moderate acne describes skin with many whiteheads, blackheads, pustules, and papules that cover one-fourth to one-half of an area. With moderate acne, the most important thing is to seek help early to prevent scarring. Your treatment regimen may include chemical peels, microdermabrasion, or blue light or red light laser therapy with ALA (see below), and/or fractional resurfacing along with skin care products.

❖ Severe acne describes deep cysts and inflammation that have caused extensive skin damage and scarring. This requires immediate treatment to prevent further damage. Treatment options are medical grade skin care products, blue light or red light laser skin rejuvenation with ALA, fractional resurfacing, and Accutane®.

❑ ALA is aminolevulinic acid, a natural substance found in your body. When combined with intense pulse light lasers or light therapies such as the LED light, it can significantly improve moderate to severe acne, including nodular cystic acne. This combination is called photodynamic therapy (PDT). PDT-ALA treatments inactivate the bacteria that trigger acne, exfoliate the skin to unclog pores, and decrease the overactive sebaceous glands in the skin that cause acne. Most patients require about three to six treatments at three to six week intervals for optimal results. Your physician will discuss this in more detail with you.

❑ Accutane® is an oral treatment for resistant acne and is very effective. Unfortunately, it has significant side effects and requires frequent monitoring with blood work. Side effects can include birth defects, liver abnormalities, depression, and severe skin dryness and night vision changes. It is used with great caution in women due to the severe teratogenic effects on the unborn fetus.

All acne treatments need to be discussed with your physician to customize them for your skin and acne severity. Eating a healthy diet, drinking water, and using good skin care products recommended by your physician will help improve your results.

PHOTOAGED/PHOTODAMAGED SKIN

Skin that has been damaged by the sun may have leathery-appearing wrinkles, excessive age spots, be dull or dry, or appear older than your biological age. At the Institute, our goal is to treat each layer of the skin to get the best rejuvenating effect for your skin. To accomplish this, we design a customized program based on a client's severity of sun damage, skin type, and budget. We usually choose a series of combination treatments with resurfacing and tightening lasers followed by injectable therapies.

As always, you must consult a skin care specialist to learn more about your options.

SUMMARY OF TREATMENT OPTIONS
FOR DIFFERENT SKIN CONDITIONS

These should be used in conjunction with good skin care products.

Skin Condition	Treatment Options
Red spots Rosacea Red skin	Laser skin rejuvenation Peels Laser vein treatments
Brown spots Acne scarring Sun damage/freckles Melasma	Microdermabrasion Peels Laser skin rejuvenation Fractional resurfacing
Acne	Peels Red light/blue light lasers ALA and light therapy Fractional resurfacing
Photo-damaged skin	Peels Microdermabrasion Laser skin rejuvenation Fractional resurfacing Laser skin tightening Injectable therapies

FINDING YOUR SKIN CARE SPECIALIST

Many people offer advanced skin care services these days, from dermatologists to plastic surgeons, primary care physicians, and medical spas. It is confusing to know where to go. I recommend doing some homework prior to any treatments.

❑ Physician training: Ask about the physician's credentials. Where were they trained and what advanced training in aesthetics have they received?

❑ Staff training: Ask who will do the service and what their training was. Many laser, microdermabrasion, and peel treatments are done by nurses and medical aestheticians. Remember there are varying degrees of training, so feel comfortable asking how many procedures they have done or supervised. Ask what the risks and benefits of the treatment are, what you should do before and after the treatment, and what complications you can expect. No matter what the service is, practitioners, if well-trained, should be able to answer these questions. If they do not know the answer, they should be able to ask a physician by phone or in person.

If the staff cannot answer these questions, they are probably not well-trained; proceed with caution. Adverse outcomes can occur even with well-trained physicians and staff, but the goal is to minimize a patient's risk with appropriate staff training and client counseling and preparation. The better informed you are, the more likely you are to make a good decision.

Our Institute provides a six-week training program for new nurses and medical aestheticians followed by a 50 percent off special for clients who go to new staff; everyone knows that the staff-person is new but trained. People get a great treatment at a great price. If I am not physically available to see someone, the staff contacts me on by phone with questions. I always try to see every person receiving a treatment somewhere in the course of treatment.

❑ Promising too much: These procedures are medical treatments that need appropriate consultation and assessment. All advanced skin care treatments work on the right type of patient. The consultation helps you learn about the treatment options but also enables the provider to see if you are a good candidate. There are no miracle treatments in this field. They will only improve, soften, blend, and refine skin; problems will not be eradicated or disappear. If this is what you are hearing or what you want, proceed with caution; you may be disappointed. Be realistic about your expectations and the results. Be specific in your questions before and after treatment.

❑ Decide if the staff listens: During the consultation, did the provider listen to your problem? What was the follow-up after your treatment? How did they respond to your questions during the consultation and any you might have afterward? You deserve to have your questions answered.

❑ Your skin type: For those with darker complexions, ask how many people of your complexion they have treated, if they have a diverse staff, and if they have literature about brown skin. Do they talk about pre-treatment conditions? Many laser companies say not to treat darker complexions, but over 40 percent of my population is some shade of olive to mahogany. We have developed techniques to help these patients with enormous success. It is important to be treated by someone who understands the needs of darker skin.

❑ Staff appearance: Lastly, does the person providing the service have good skin? I can't tell you how important this is. If the provider does not have great skin, then they are not practicing what they preach. How can you be assured that these treatments work? When I started, I did not have great skin. I explained to every client what I was doing to help my acne and scarring. I could show before and after pictures of the improvements you can see with good skin care products and treatments. My story was real, and my patients appreciated it.

HAIR REMOVAL: LASER HAIR REMOVAL, ELECTROLYSIS, AND THREADING

Hair removal of any sort is still one of the most sought-after cosmetic services. Permanent hair reduction with lasers can be done on all skin types and anywhere on the body. Laser hair removal takes about six to ten visits. The more hair you have, the longer it will take. The darker your skin is, the more treatments you will require because the laser has to be at a lower setting to protect the skin from hyperpigmentation. Laser hair removal will only permanently reduce hair growth about 70 to 80 percent on light skin and 60 to 70 percent on brown skin. There is no such thing as 100 percent hair removal. Laser hair removal does not work on grey, white, or blond hair.

If you do not see a result, speak with your physician to see if you may have a hormonal problem or need to try a more aggressive laser hair removal treatment. As always, you need to discuss with your physician to determine if you are a good candidate for laser hair removal, what results you can expect, and if any pretreatment is necessary.

With laser hair removal able to treat large areas faster and cheaper, electrolysis has become less popular. I still recommend it for people with light hair, fine hair, or just a few hairs in an area.

Hair can also be removed with waxing or threading. Threading is an ancient Indian and Persian technique to remove unwanted facial hair using just a cotton thread. This technique provides such a precise shape to the eyebrows that once people have done threading, most will never use another method! I like threading as a complement to medical spas because it is not a contraindication to any treatment like waxing is. More importantly, clients using Retin-A do not have to stop it for hair removal.

BUILDING SPOKE SIX
OF YOUR PERSONAL WELLNESS WHEEL™

❑ Examine your life to see if you can eliminate or reduce any extrinsic aging effects on your skin, such as sun exposure or exposure to cigarette smoke.

❑ Use a broad-spectrum sunblock daily, whether you plan to be indoors or outdoors, to protect your skin from UVA and UVB rays.

❑ Visit a skin care professional to determine the best skin care products for your skin type and age. Remember that using products to PREVENT future problems is much easier and inexpensive than fixing problems once they occur.

❑ Complete the "Ageless Skin Chart" on page 127 to determine what skin concerns you might like to address.

❑ Research your options for skin care treatments. Using the "finding your skin care specialist" section on pages 123-124, prepare a list of questions to ask when you contact or visit a potential facility. Be sure they give you adequate answers! Remember that you have choices and that finding a knowledgeable and qualified skin care professional is among the most important.

❑ Drink plenty of water to hydrate your skin; reduce your alcohol consumption.

❑ Find and determine the factors of your appearance that make you proud and happy; focusing on these will give you confidence to move toward overall Optimal Health.

AGELESS SKIN CHART

Name:_____ Age: _____ Date:_____

Complete this chart by filling in your skin concerns. After meeting with your skin care specialist, record the different treatments recommended. The column "Skin Goals" is what you hope to achieve from the treatments as well as how much improvement your skin care specialist stated you would have. In the last column, you can track your progress with the different treatments.

Skin Concerns	Types of Treatments	Skin Goals	Improvement from Treatment(s)

We must be the change we wish to see.

~ Mohandas Gandhi

Spoke Seven

STRESS MANAGEMENT TECHNIQUES: BALANCING YOUR MIND AND BODY

CONTENTS:
* the effects of stress on your body
* risk factors of stress
* how to handle stress effectively
* the benefits of meditation
* changing your mind
* building spoke seven

Stress management is an important part of your Personal Wellness Wheel™. In Eastern philosophy, the mind and body are inter-related. No matter how well you are progressing with the other spokes of the wheel, if you are unable to manage your stress, you will have much more difficulty reaching your goal of Optimal Health. Remember, Optimal Health requires synergy and integration of all the elements of the Personal Wellness Wheel™. When you start practicing the stress management techniques presented here, you will see the benefits—and realize that you can effectively deal with the stress in your job, your life, and yourself.

In this chapter, you will learn the following:
- ○ The Effects of Stress on Your Body
- ○ Risk Factors of Stress
- ○ How to Handle Stress Effectively
- ○ The Benefits of Meditation
- ○ Changing Your Mind

THE EFFECTS OF STRESS ON YOUR BODY

Stress is the body's general response to change. It can have both positive and negative effects, depending on the amount of stress and the perceived control we have over the stressor (change). Your personal stress level depends on many factors, including your personality, your general outlook on life, your problem-solving abilities, and your social support system.

For example, some people do well under "stress" because they get more work done, especially when they are on a deadline. This positive benefit can occur because of the increased energy your body produces to help you meet a challenge. For example, getting married or having a baby are usually positive changes for most people, but are still stressors because they involve change.

However, when a stressor becomes chronic, more intense, or if we perceive we have less control over it, it can become a negative. This type of stress may lead to many different medical conditions.

Your initial physiologic response to stress is a surge in cortisol and adrenaline. This is not harmful. In fact, it is protective because it allows you to prepare. But frequent, prolonged surges of the cortisol response can lead to many health problems, including:

❖ Elevated blood sugar (glucose), which over time can increase your risk for diabetes. High levels of glucose can increase cholesterol production, which further increases your risk for heart disease.

- ❖ Higher insulin levels as a response to increased blood sugar. Insulin is the hormone that puts blood sugar into your muscles. As we learned in the nutrition spoke (Chapter Three), elevated levels of insulin cause increases in body fat, especially in the midsection. The heavier your midsection is, the greater your resistance to insulin, which then further increases weight gain. Extra body fat also increases your risk for heart disease and slows the release of growth hormone, the master hormone that helps us stay young.
- ❖ Increased blood pressure. High blood pressure over time increases your risk for heart disease.
- ❖ Increased silent inflammation (which accelerates the aging process).
- ❖ Decreased immunity.
- ❖ Decreases in sleep. When you sleep less, your body does not get a chance to recover. Poor sleep has been associated with poor eating habits, leading you to eat higher glycemic foods, further increasing your blood sugar and insulin levels and beginning an out-of-control spiral. Poor sleep also leads to a decline in your natural production of growth hormone. This further causes you to age faster and degenerate; lower growth hormone levels are associated with increasing body fat, decreasing muscle mass, insulin resistance, poor cognitive affects, loss of memory, lower libido, lowered immunity, and sexual dysfunction.

To summarize, the negative effects of stress can affect the progress of your Personal Wellness Wheel™ by affecting nutrition, decreasing your desire to exercise, affecting your body's natural production of hormones, and increasing silent inflammation which worsens chronic disease and can accelerate the aging process.

THE SYMPTOMS OF STRESS

Symptoms of stress can be broken down into the physical, cognitive (mental), behavioral, and emotional. Circle the number of symptoms you have on each list below and write your total on the table on page 133 to measure the number of stressors in your life. The more you have, the worse your ability to handle stress.

The Physical Symptoms of Stress

- Chest pain
- Weight gain or loss
- Frequent colds
- Chronic pain
- High blood pressure
- Headaches/migraines
- Indigestion/ulcers
- Stomachaches
- Sweaty palms
- Sleep difficulties
- Heart disease
- Diabetes
- Asthma
- PMS
- Obesity
- Tiredness
- Loss of libido
- Diarrhea or constipation
- Insomnia
- Low sperm count
- Infertility
- Autoimmune diseases
- Irritable bowel syndrome
- Skin problems (acne, wrinkles)
- Dizziness
- Back pain
- Tight neck and shoulders
- Racing heart
- Restlessness

The Cognitive Symptoms of Stress

- Trouble thinking clearly
- Lack of creativity
- Inability to make decisions
- Inability to concentrate
- Seeing only negatives in life
- Fearfulness
- Forgetfulness
- Memory loss
- Constant worry
- Poor judgment
- Loss of objectivity

The Behavioral Symptoms of Stress

- Excessive smoking
- Compulsive gum chewing
- Grinding your teeth at night
- Compulsive eating or not eating
- Overdoing activities such as exercise or shopping
- Over-reacting to unexpected problems
- Bossiness
- An attitude critical of others
- Overuse of alcohol
- Inability to get things done
- Sleeping too much or too little

The Emotional Symptoms of Stress

- ❖ Crying
- ❖ Anxiety
- ❖ Edginess (a readiness to explode)
- ❖ An overwhelming sense of pressure
- ❖ Easily upset
- ❖ Depression

- ❖ Nervousness
- ❖ Loneliness
- ❖ Feeling powerless to change things
- ❖ Boredom (finding no meaning in anything)
- ❖ Moodiness

Cumulative Effects

Now add up your total stressors in each category.

Symptoms	Your score	Minimal	Moderate	Severe
Physical		≤ 10	11-15	≥ 16
Cognitive		≤ 2	3-5	≥ 6
Emotional		≤ 2	3-5	≥ 6
Behavioral		≤ 2	3-5	≥ 6
Total		≤ 16	17-27	≥ 28

People's stress manifests differently. Some people have more physical symptoms, some have more emotional, and others have all of them. Use this test to help you understand how you react to stress, both small and big. That way you can begin to manage stress before it becomes overwhelming.

RISK FACTORS OF STRESS

What are the sources of stress? Major life changes are very stressful; the more you have at one time, the worse your stress will be.

MOST STRESSFUL LIFE EVENTS

TOP TEN MOST STRESSFUL LIFE EVENTS

❖ Spouse's death
❖ Divorce
❖ Marriage separation
❖ Jail term
❖ Death of a close relative

❖ Injury or illness
❖ Marriage
❖ Being fired from job
❖ Marriage reconciliation
❖ Retirement

Source: Holmes-Rahe Life Stress Inventory.
See the appendix (pp. 170-171) for the full list.

To this top-ten list, I add any traumatic experience that causes grief and loss, such as experiencing or witnessing a crime, natural disaster, losing a loved one to violence, or violence at school or work.

But for most of us, it is the daily challenges that are stressful. These stressors can be divided into:

❖ Family and relationship stressors: difficulties with our family members, friends, or romantic partners, as well as caring for chronically-ill family members can cause stress.

❖ Work stressors: Work stress can be caused by job dissatisfaction, an increased workload, insufficient pay, office politics, and conflicts with your boss or co-workers.

❖ Social stressors: Your social situation (such as financial difficulties or pressures, racial and sexual discrimination, unemployment, isolation, or a lack of social support) can cause stress.

❖ Environmental stressors: Your physical surroundings can set off the stress response. Examples of environmental stressors include an unsafe neighborhood, pollution, noise (sirens keeping you up at night, a barking dog next door), and uncomfortable living conditions.

Internal Causes of Stress

Outside of the external causes are internal stressors pertaining to our abilities and tendencies such as:

- ❖ Uncertainty or worries
- ❖ A pessimistic attitude
- ❖ Self-criticism
- ❖ Unrealistic expectations
- ❖ Perfectionism
- ❖ Low self-esteem
- ❖ Excessive or unexpressed anger
- ❖ A lack of assertiveness

These internal behaviors or reactions can increase stress. They are often rooted in our childhood experiences and can be addressed once you recognize that you need to change how you handle stress. Try the recommendations suggested here to see if they can help you deal with your stress more effectively. If you are having difficulty reframing your thoughts, you may want to seek the help of a psychotherapist to help you. Remember that many of your attitudes may change once you put your Personal Wellness Wheel™ into practice.

HOW TO HANDLE STRESS EFFECTIVELY

Stress is inevitable; your task is to manage it. Here are three key ideas to help handle your stress.

❑ How important is it?
❑ What can you do about it?
❑ What can you let go?

When confronted with a stressful situation, ask yourself these questions and write down the answers using the following guidelines:

❑ First, ask yourself: How important is it? Everything is important, but some things are more important. Rank this stress event from 1 to 10. Now that you have a number, ask yourself how important it is with regard to your entire life. Now rate the event again. The purpose of this question is to make the event more manageable. Many events can be seen as a 2 or a 5. Rating something a 9 means that the event is truly life-changing, such as a death in your family or a catastrophe. A marriage is a life-changing event, but not usually of the catastrophic category!

❑ Next, ask yourself the second question: What can I do about it? Use the following guide:

- ■ What I can change
- ■ What cannot be changed
- ■ What I have to accept

This is crucially important because nearly any situation has things which you can change, things which you cannot, and things which you must accept. What can you change about the stressful situation? Is there anything you can do to improve it? Determine what you absolutely cannot change and strive toward acceptance on that issue.

❑ Finally, the third question is, what can I let go? After answering the first two questions, you may find this easier. Often, we need to let go of the outcome. We cannot control how things turn out; we can only prepare ourselves in the best way possible. We can let go of anxiety and fearfulness and concentrate on our self-confidence.

❑ Here is an example to help you: Jason has an important meeting at 9 AM. He knows he will have to convince the majority of people to accept his ideas. His performance rating depends on how well the meeting goes. He knows there will be resistance to his ideas. His anxiety about the meeting is causing stress. Let's use the formula presented above:

- ■ "How important is the stress event?" On a scale of 1 to 10, Jason places it at a 5. This helps because in his mind his feelings of stress have placed it at a 10. He realizes that while it is very important, it is not a 10. In the total scheme of his life, it is important, but it is only a meeting. This helps Jason to scale down his stress so that he can manage it.
- ■ "What can I do about it?" Jason determines that the best thing he can do is prepare well for the meeting and boost his confidence. He can stop worrying about everyone else and focus on his abilities. He reviews his presentation. He improves it or leaves it as it is.
- ■ "What can I let go?" Jason must let go of his focus on the outcome. He must focus instead on preparing himself in the best way possible for the meeting. He needs to develop his confidence, his presentation, and his abilities. He may not be able to change the way everyone thinks and may have to accept that some people might not like his ideas. He concludes that he can only do his best and cannot control the outcome.

This exercise demonstrates an important principle of stress management: cutting the stress down to size and controlling the aspects you can. In high stress situations, the stress appears overwhelming; using this exercise will help you master it.

STRESS MANAGEMENT EXERCISE

Define the event.
❑ Rate its stress level: 1 to 10 scale
❑ What can I do about it?
■ what can I change?
■ what can't I change?
■ what do I have to accept?
❑ What can I let go?

THE BENEFITS OF MEDITATION

One of the most powerful tools for stress management is meditation. It can help you develop composure and a clear mind. Neuroscientists have shown that meditation shifts brain activity from the stress-prone right frontal cortex to the left frontal cortex; the result is less anxiety and depression. Research has also shown that meditators have less activity in the brain's amygdala, which controls fear; therefore, meditation can help you deal with fears. Meditation states are the same as those that occur during deep sleep, so this may help release growth hormone naturally! Other benefits of meditation are that it

❖ Slows heart rate
❖ Lowers blood pressure
❖ Calms metabolic and respiratory systems
❖ Lowers stress and anxiety response
❖ Enhances perceptual ability
❖ Improves focus and concentration
❖ Helps control chronic anxiety.

Meditation is simply a pause from the busy world you live in. It allows you to deeply relax and suspend the active thought process. It creates a state of being, rather than one of "doing." Through daily practice, you will begin to see a change in the way you handle stress.

PROPER BREATHING

Before you begin any meditation practice, it is important to focus on your breathing. Most of us are shallow breathers. We need to learn how to breathe!

Here is an exercise to practice:

A BREATHING EXERCISE

Sitting up straight in your chair, put your feet on the ground and your hands in your lap. Begin by taking a long, slow, steady breath in through your nose. Pause for a second, and then exhale slowly through your mouth.

Try this again, concentrating on your breath. See if you can draw your breath into your chest and even your stomach. Practice this exercise ten times. Notice how you feel. Are you able to feel your breath and where it moves in your body?

You may notice you feel calmer. Notice, too, that your breathing can be much deeper than your normal shallow breath.

Practice this every day. The goal is to make this your normal breath and to stop shallow breathing. Make it a habit: every time you feel stressed, stop and practice your breathing. It can make a difference.

MODERN MEDITATION TECHNIQUE

Many types of meditation are available; some resources are listed in the appendix. I use a simple method called Modern Meditation. I have found it easy to learn and accessible for busy people who need stress relief. I recommend beginning your meditation practice at home, preferably in the morning. Although everyone is busy in the morning, the benefits you achieve will be worth it.

Set aside fifteen minutes (five minutes for each step) to practice the three steps outlined below. Choose a quiet place and a comfortable chair. Loosen any clothing and place your feet firmly on the ground and your hands in your lap. Begin any mediation you choose by practicing your breathing exercise.

MODERN MEDITATION TECHNIQUE

Step One: Relaxing the Body (five minutes)

This step relieves tension and stress in your body. By practicing a "body scan" (which takes about five minutes), you can easily learn to push out the tension in your body, starting at the top of your head and moving slowly to your feet. The goal is to deeply relax to prepare for step two.

Step Two: Calming the Mind (five minutes)

This step will help quiet your busy mind. Our minds are full of chatter, worry, and anxiety. These are only thoughts and need to be controlled, so that we can experience deep quiet. When we suspend our thoughts, we can truly relax and create a space for new, creative, and useful thoughts.

Step Three: Freeing the Spirit (five minutes)

This step is designed to help you locate and identify the peaceful, creative space within. With practice, you gain a way of accessing this "location" easily and quickly, wherever you are.

This simple method can be practiced like a "power nap" whenever your thoughts or stress become overwhelming. You can take a break, practice your breathing, and do the three steps quickly and effectively. Remember, the more you practice, the more it will become second nature.

At first, you may only be able to practice for fifteen minutes, but later you may find you are able to practice for longer periods of time, enhancing the health benefits.

A complete guide to this exercise is on page 141.

RELAXATION

Relaxation techniques are similar to meditation but are not as formal. We recommend that you build time for relaxation into your schedule, no matter how busy it is. Without effective forms of relaxation, you cannot recharge yourself, balance work and life, and achieve Optimal Health.

There are many forms of relaxation. Here are a few:

❖ Walking
❖ Sports
❖ Hobbies
❖ Music

❖ Art
❖ Reading
❖ Nature
❖ Anything that brings you joy!

CHANGING YOUR MIND

As a result of changing your breathing patterns and practicing meditation, you will find that you can "change your mind." This means that you will be able to recognize your thinking patterns and change them at will.

Identifying your thinking is necessary before you can change it. The following example will help you understand this exercise:

CHANGING YOUR MIND EXERCISE

1. Identify the thought:
Example: I am thinking that the project I have to do is tedious and too hard.

2. What kind of thought is it?
Example: Negative

3. What can I change about my thinking?
Example: Find something good about the project.

This is a simple yet effective way to begin the process of change. You can train your mind to work for you instead of against you.

CREATING JOY

In our day-to-day lives, most of us are so busy that we may not engage in activities that bring us joy. Every person has activities that bring happiness and satisfaction. We need to try to do these activities on a regular basis to alleviate some stress. If you do not know what creates joy in your life, take time now to list (on the sheet provided on page 142) ten things that help you feel better or bring peace to you. Now try to schedule something in your life—minimally once per week—to do something from your list.

The last comment on creating joy is giving. Practicing compassion and giving are wonderful sources of creating joy that can provide deep peace. I recommend that each of us volunteer in some way to help our community. This act of giving to others makes us more grateful for what we have and provides a way to improve our communities.

BUILDING SPOKE SEVEN
OF YOUR PERSONAL WELLNESS WHEEL™

☐ Review the effects of stress and make a list of your stress symptoms.

☐ List your risk factors from the Holmes-Rahe Life Stress Inventory on pages 170-171.

☐ Use the following exercise to handle stress effectively whenever you need it.
- ❖ Define the event and rate the stress on a scale of 1 to 10.
- ❖ What can you do about it?
  - ♦ what can you change?
  - ♦ what can't you change?
  - ♦ what do you have to accept?
- ❖ What can you let go?

☐ Practice the breathing exercise several times a day or whenever needed: Sitting up straight in your chair, put your feet on the ground and your hands in your lap. Begin by taking a long, slow, steady breath in through your nose. Pause for a second, and then exhale slowly through your mouth. Try this again, concentrating on your breath. See if you can draw your breath into your chest and even your stomach. Practice until your breathing is steady and calm.

☐ Meditation Practice: Once a day for a minimum of fifteen minutes. Begin by closing your eyes and practicing the breathing exercise.

- ❖ Step One, Relaxing the Body: Imagine that you are pushing your stress down, from head to toe. Start at the top of your head and gradually move toward your feet, scanning your shoulders, neck, arms, stomach, hips, legs, slowly pushing the tension down as you go, until finally, you reach your feet. Imagine the stress flowing out of your feet and into the ground, where you let it go. Remember to breathe deeply as you push downward.

- ❖ Step Two, Calming the Mind: Now imagine that you can quiet your busy mind. When a thought comes to you, simply guide the thought out of your mindspace. Acknowledge the thought and say that you will consider it later, after meditation. Repeat with each thought that arises: simply guide it out of your mindspace. Remember to breathe deeply as each thought leaves.

- ❖ Step Three, Freeing the Spirit: Renew your spirit by locating a special place within yourself that is calm, creative, and free. It is the infinite space, where your thoughts disappear and you can access peace and calm. Try at first to imagine a special place that you identify as your own. Each time you practice mediation, you can return there.

Remember, meditation is a life-long practice. It requires allowing yourself to set aside time to practice. If at first you don't succeed, keep trying!

❑ Changing Your Mind: Use the following exercise several times, until it becomes a habit.
  ❖ Identify your thought.
  ❖ What kind of thought is it?
  ❖ What can I do to change my thinking?
❑ Relaxation Techniques: Build time for relaxation into your schedule, no matter how busy it is. Without effective forms of relaxation, you cannot recharge yourself, balance your work and life, or achieve Optimal Health. Find ways that work for you.

ACTIVITIES THAT HELP ME RELAX

Spoke Eight

YOUR STRATEGIES FOR SUCCESS: CHOOSING YOUR PATH WISELY

What we think, we become.
~ Buddha

Written by Lee Kirksey, MD.

CONTENTS:
* motivation for change:
the "why" question
* the force behind change
* either you guide your
associations or someone else will
* the optimistic personality
and health
* optimism and optimal health

One of my great joys in life is practicing medicine. Despite the tremendous tide of change sweeping across the field of healthcare, I feel genuinely blessed for a number of reasons. Despite a number of opinion polls describing the waning level of regard and respect for doctors and healthcare, I think that most people really like "their physician." It's human nature to have an almost inevitable emotion of gratitude after another human being has helped you.

Secondly, I believe that the patient-doctor relationship is the most precious of interactions between two human beings. Many professionals can interact with people on a group level to convey a general message. For example, a minister can talk to a congregation and effectively communicate her message. A teacher can talk to his class to teach a lesson. But by and large, no matter how much technology advances, for the moment the doctor solves problems one patient at a time. A relationship is developed. Information is exchanged and recommendations are extended. The trust that is necessary for that process to work effectively is beyond belief. And as a person who receives this level of trust, thousands of time per year, I frequently marvel at the responsibility.

As a surgeon, the privilege to accurately diagnose illness and then offer a treatment that corrects the process, sometimes immediately, is awe-inspiring. The technology that we use in operations to treat patients has evolved significantly in a short period of time. In many cases, we can now actually "sneak" into the body with a minimally invasive procedure to treat a disease with much less trauma to the patient.

One of the most frequent questions people ask me is what type of medications they should take to decrease their risks of heart attack or stroke; younger people ask me what type of diet they should be on to prevent blockages from developing. These are great questions. To the second, I generally respond that I dislike the word "diet." Just the thought of it, in my opinion, represents a process of struggle and sacrifice. I really don't perceive "diet" as a long-term strategy with a high chance of sustainability.

This underscores a major premise of the Optimal Health Program. The Optimal Health Program is about long-term, sustainable lifestyle changes. It is an integrated strategy to identify core areas of emphasis as a fundamental basis upon which to develop and improve. There are strategies for success in this quest.

Spoke Eight, "Your Strategies for Success," was written by Lee Kirksey, MD.

In this chapter, you will learn the following:
- Motivation for Change: The "Why" Question
- The Force Behind Change
- Either You Guide Your Associations or Someone Else Will
- The Optimistic Personality and Health
- Optimism and Optimal Health

MOTIVATION FOR CHANGE: THE "WHY" QUESTION

The motivation to make health changes is present in all of us. But we must call upon and focus this motivation in the right direction. The motivation to change begins with creating what I refer to as a strong "why" question. "Why" is what drives apparently "average" people to achieve beyond what appears "realistic" to others. It may result in a fantastic story like a high school dropout named Dave Thomas who opens a restaurant that would someday be an international franchise named Wendy's. It could be a high school basketball player cut from the varsity squad as a sophomore who consistently improves his skills until he ultimately becomes arguably the world's best basketball player. On a different level, it could be the mom who wants to get into better shape and arises at 5 AM to work out for an hour before the rest of her family awakens just so she can enjoy the fruits of good health as her children age.

My point is that the why question is the primary driving force behind any change. And the more vivid and visceral your idea is, the more likely you are to complete the action. Consider: When was the last time you were briefly inspired to lose a couple of pounds because you wanted to fit into that special outfit? You dieted, gave up your favorite candy, walked at lunch. Maybe you wore the fantastic, form-fitting dress to the organization dinner, class reunion, or wedding. If you're like most people, you proceeded to gain the lost weight back in the subsequent weeks or months. The "why" was gone. Short-term, transient goals. Short-term results. Why do *you* want Optimal Health?

DEVELOPING YOUR "WHY" LIST

To develop your "why" list, sit alone quietly and use the meditative routine found in Spoke Seven. Then list compelling reasons why an overall program for improved health is beneficial to you, as an individual or part of a group or organization. Think of it as circles of influence that increase progressively.

Example:

1. If I were healthier, I would have more energy for work and time with my family.
2. If I were healthier, my self-image would improve.
3. If my preventative health strategies were optimized, I would have the best chance of watching my children grow into adulthood and have their own children (my grandchildren).
4. If I avoid or minimize chronic disease, I would be able to enjoy my retirement years with travel and a great quality of life. I might be able to avoid the loss of quality time that accompanies the intense medical requirement of chronic disease states.
5. If I were healthier, I might avoid or minimize the chronic disease that is the largest post-retirement expense for most older Americans.
6. As a role model for my children, strong life management skills are among the best tools that I could possibly create.
7. Many healthy habits are established early and would be better received early in my children's lives.

THE FORCE BEHIND CHANGE

The force behind change is very basic in origin. Whether we take an action is primarily driven by our need to avoid pain and our desire to maximize pleasure. We frequently voice a desire to make changes in our lives, but whether we will depends on these factors.

Why haven't you returned to the dentist yet? You know that you should. You have had cavities in the past, and they may have recurred. But you still haven't made an appointment for a checkup. It is because in your mind the inconvenience of scheduling, rearranging your schedule, and driving to the appointment is more prominent than the pain you associate with a developing cavity. The former is real in your perception, while the latter is unlikely. You rationalize that you just went to the dentist a year ago, and the likelihood of the dentist actually finding a cavity is quite small. In this quick moment your subconscious leads you to believe that the dentist appointment can wait.

This field of study is named neuro-associative conditioning, the process that usually takes place subconsciously and drives our decision-making. The field is broad and too extensive to explain in its entirety here, but I will introduce some of its basic concepts. Hopefully, it will explain some of the "behind the scenes" activity that occurs when we are on "autopilot." In my opinion, our ability to effectively recognize and control our neuro-associations is the cornerstone of implementing intentional, sustainable change: not change that just happens by chance, but change that is predictable and under your control.

I have no doubt that if you're reading this book, you are a highly motivated person interested in improving your life. Not that your life is not already fine. But I suspect that you would like to use the Optimal Health Program to have an extraordinary life experience. Neuro-associative training and conditioning are essential to implementing the core preventative health, lifestyle changes, nutrition, exercise, hormonal modulation, advanced skincare therapies, and stress management of your Personal Wellness Wheel™.

The first task is to recognize our neuro-associations and to understand how they motivate us for change or stagnation. Let me share some of mine. I associate a tremendous amount of pleasure with being physically fit. I have played sports all of my life, and it's very important that I maintain a constant level of conditioning. Similarly, I associate a lot of pain with anything that contributes to poor conditioning like smoking, overeating, or extended periods of not exercising. I also place a very high value on learning. Not just knowing a lot of facts, but being able to teach myself new ideas and topics and subsequently being able to share with and teach others. You can see how these neuro-associations would influence me to stay late after work, get up early before work, and forgo vacations to write and finish this book with Dr. Patel. Neuro-associations are powerful moderators of behavior. When chosen wisely, they can lead to very positive changes in your life and can be a compass to guide your direction of growth.

On the other hand, I also developed a very bad neuro-association early in my life while playing sports. Early in my childhood, I experienced a great deal of success in various sports like baseball and basketball. I began to associate a great deal of pleasure with winning. My child's mind noticed that everyone—other kids, teachers, parents—likes a winner. People seemed to treat me differently when I won. My family even changed our vacation based upon when a playoff would occur. It really became very important to win. Of course, nothing is wrong with desiring to win. Competition is healthy and makes all involved better. But I think the better, more helpful neuro-association would have been to never quit and to give 110 percent effort on each occasion: less emphasis on the outcome and more emphasis on the process of effort. As we all know, if you practice diligently and perform with great effort, you are likely to have a good outcome. As a result of this focus on winning, I developed a great fear of the opposite alternative: losing. And when you begin to excessively fear losing and the potential of failing, you lose your focus and begin to paradoxically perform worse. I began to see myself putting forth more effort . . . only to get worse outcomes. And the more you think about something, the less fluid your thoughts and motions are, especially in tasks that require rapid, instinctual responses like sports. Fortunately, I was able to identify this underlying process and return some balance to my neuro-associations.

In the current phase of my life, training surgical residents, from time to time I see signs of the "fear of failure." I now know how to manage it for myself and how to assist others in learning how to manage it for themselves. It is not an overstatement to say that the associations that you develop at a young age and over the course of your life can shape your ultimate destiny.

NEURO-ASSOCIATIONS AND YOUR HEALTH

What kind of neuro-associations do you have about your health and well-being? It's important to realize that many of our neuro-associations are subconscious. We don't even think of them. They are vast accumulations of experiences over our lifetime. Some are from your childhood, reinforced by family, friends, and cultural beliefs. Some are reinforced by trial and error over time. These neuro-associations sometimes masquerade under the headings of "values," "principles," and "beliefs." Whatever word you use to represent these ideas, work hard to introspect and uncover them. Only then will you be able to sort out what's helpful and what's harmful as you work toward Optimal Health.

I would like you to make two lists. List One will consist of positive health behaviors. I want you to group these under whether you associate them with pleasure or pain. (See below.) In List Two, you will do the same thing for what you perceive to be negative behaviors. Be honest or it won't help you. Obviously, you will have some perceived negative behaviors that provide you with some pleasure and some perceived positive behaviors that you associate with pain.

List One: Positive Health Behaviors	Associated with Pain	Associated with Pleasure
	going to dentist	exercising three times weekly
	dieting	dieting
List Two: Negative Health Behaviors	**Associated with Pain**	**Associated with Pleasure**
	smoking	ice cream and cookies

The next part of this exercise is to determine the events that influenced these beliefs. I personally had a very painful experience with a dentist as a child. To this day, I am very untrusting of dentists. This certainly has influenced the frequency of my return to the dentist.

Finally, make a list of five to ten life-changing actions, such as starting an exercise program, reading one new book per month, enrolling in an online course, reconnecting with a lost friend or relative, or taking a stress management class. Think about all the negative consequences that may occur as a result of not following through on these actions. Visualize the consequences very descriptively and viscerally; I want you to feel something as you describe the negative impact: no sugar coating. Dig deep.

EITHER YOU GUIDE YOUR ASSOCIATIONS OR SOMEONE ELSE WILL

How does this neuro-association play a role in your behavior overall? The value of neuro-associations has been recognized for years. Look at an obvious example: the constant barrage of advertisements on TV, radio, in print, and now on the internet.

Think about your favorite song from high school—the one that, every time you hear it, brings you back to a moment in time when you were carefree, lacked worries, and had the energy and optimism of youth. Maybe it was Bruce Springstein or Michael Jackson's "Thriller." You know what song it was for you. Now attach that song to an image of your favorite fancy car. Maybe it's a convertible or a nice sedan. If the song provokes intense enough emotion and you associate it with a visual of the cherished car, soon you will begin to associate the provoked emotion with the automobile. It's the same trick advertisers have used for years: find an emotionally provocative person (spokesmodel), image, or song and tie it to the product they want you to desire. Neuro-association in action. My point is that if you don't control your neuro-associations, plenty of advertising products vying for the attention and consumer dollars of you and your family will fill that role.

Here is a perfect example that I find fascinating because I know what the trick is, but despite my resistance, it influences how I feel. Some commercials make it look so fun to drink a lot of alcohol and eat a lot of greasy food that they almost make me forget that I barely like the taste of either. Alcohol gives me an excruciating headache, it interferes with my sleep, and I'm tired for forty-eight hours after. Greasy food gives me an upset stomach and diarrhea, and I know that I have to ride the treadmill fast for twenty minutes to burn 150 calories (one slice of bread). Whose neuro-association and belief will serve you better if you want to resist the temptation of the commercial and avoid the empty calories of liquor and the excess calories of a large, greasy meal?

THE OPTIMISTIC PERSONALITY AND HEALTH

We are beginning to see that if we want to be successful at working toward Optimal Health, we need to be in control. How do our personalities fit into this? The role that individual personality plays in our abilities to defend our bodies against illness has been a subject of much debate for many years. Let's imagine two people with the same type of cancer at the same stage of progression. All their other health factors are identical, including age and additional medical conditions. One individual manages to avoid depression and survive for several years following the initial diagnosis while the other person, immediately upon receiving news of the illness, falls into a deep depression and despite all efforts, seems to "give up," dying within several months of the initial diagnosis.

In my practice dealing with cardiovascular patients, I have always believed that an extraordinarily optimistic personality causes some people to deal much better with adversity. This belief is held by many others and supported with anecdotal experiences and patient stories. Accumulating medical information is substantiating many such claims about the mind and body connection in defending the body against illness.

Medical literature seems to support several facts about this relationship:

❖ Optimists have better health maintenance habits compared to pessimists.
❖ Optimism seems to promote immune system competence.
❖ People with optimistic personalities tend to live longer than pessimists.
❖ Optimists suffer a fewer number of infections.

STYLE OF EXPLAINING LIFE EVENTS

If your personality does impact your health over the course of your lifetime, how can this influence be rationally explained? Dr. Martin Seligman, a well-known psychologist at the University of Pennsylvania, theorized that a person's ability to behave as an optimist or pessimist is largely dependent upon his or her style of explaining life events.

Suppose you have made an internal commitment to a pattern of healthy eating habits. Colleagues invite you to an after-work event on a beautiful Friday afternoon. You accept, but remind yourself that you are on a diet and plan to stick to your guns. After a while, the revelry of the evening begins to influence you; you have your favorite calorie-laden tropical cocktail, followed by a host of appetizers such as nachos with cheese, calamari, and other fried fats. You complete the evening by joining the group in eating cheesecake. When you arrive home, you realize that you have violated your personal commitment to healthy eating.

Dr. Seligman posits that how you explain this event to yourself will ultimately determine how you respond to this challenge. You could choose the explanation that you don't have any control over your eating habits, that you always give in to temptation, and that you know that's the way it will always be. This permanent, pervasive, and personal way of describing this negative Friday-evening event will cause an ongoing sense of helplessness. If you describe it as a temporary lapse—"it was just one evening and as long as I resume my habits tomorrow, I haven't done much damage; I can recover"—or nonpervasive—"I usually am very disciplined; this was a unique lapse; if I have a 'cheat day' once a month, the world won't come to a halt"—you are likely to recover uneventfully, with only a brief period of helplessness and your self-image intact.

The second way that the presence of optimistic personality characteristics leads to good health is in how we perceive our control over our own health. Consider a person who has a negative, pessimistic internal explanation of healthcare maintenance. She perceives medical illness as pervasive, permanent, and personal: "Nothing that I can do makes a difference, so why bother to change?" This person is more likely to continue smoking, not exercising, undertaking unsafe and risky health behaviors, and not participating in appropriate health screenings for preventable and treatable medical illnesses (such as flu vaccination, mammography for breast cancer, pap smear for cervical cancer, and colonoscopy for colon cancer). This person is less likely to have routine recommended doctor's visits and less likely to follow a doctor's recommendations for treatment. This person is unlikely to visit a doctor until advanced symptoms of disease develop.

Here is an example. Once I worked with a very bright young nurse in my hospital. She had excelled in her nursing training and by all accounts was very capable in providing patient care. I always saw her congregated with a group in the designated smoking area outside the hospital. Several times I made brief, facetious comments suggesting how I felt about smoking and how surprised I was to see her amongst the smokers. It's always sad to me to see people, shivering in the midst of winter and huddled in a small confined area, smoking cigarettes. It really defines the physically and psychologically addictive nature of nicotine.

I always tell people that if you see a problem and choose to ignore it, you're probably part of the problem. And if you see a friend with a problem and choose to say nothing, are you genuinely a friend? So I asked her one day, "With all you know, having seen lung surgeries for cancer and having seen tracheostomies for throat cancer, how can you continue to smoke?" She said, embarrassed, "I know, I really should have tried to stop several times." She acknowledged several of my attempts to perform some brief neuro-associative conditioning. I vividly described the smell smoke creates on the body, clothes, and home, its effect on the teeth, and the loss of exercise capacity.

What followed was quite interesting. She described how her father had recently died at a relatively young age from an advanced abdominal cancer. He became symptomatic and was diagnosed immediately, dying within six months of the onset of symptoms. Obviously a very stressful time in her life, she began to smoke more. Additionally, she had a grandmother who "smoked like a chimney" and lived until the age of 93. What she was describing to me was a very subtle line of thinking that obviously led her to conclude that your life behaviors don't matter. Very compelling life experiences had reinforced for her that lifestyle and illness development are not connected. I concluded that my apparently rational explanation of why she should stop smoking would not be adequate to change her strong perceptions about cause and effect.

I think that this is one of the primary areas in which physicians, healthcare professionals, and public policymakers fail in our attempts to change behaviors which create illnesses. We explain things to people in ways that make sense to us, not accounting for the fact that their realities may be different from ours.

Unfortunately, from time to time in training and in practice, I have seen a patient who presented with some disease whose physical manifestations were obviously visible, such as an externally protruding mass on the breast or a gangrenous and foul-smelling body part. Before I learned about explanation style and learned helplessness, I had an extremely difficult time understanding this circumstance and why someone would wait so long before addressing this type of medical concern. Now, I recognize that this characteristic differs (to some degree) from denial. Many times, people in denial act as if something does not exist. In contrast, with an explanation style of learned helplessness, a person fully acknowledges the problem, but through life experiences, has concluded that rectifying the problem is impossible.

In a study of pessimism and its effect on health, patients were tested for their level of cynicism, defeatism, and pessimism. They received information about steps to prevent medical illness and screening tests for early diagnosis of medical disease. The most pessimistic people spent the least amount of time reviewing the material and had the worst recall of details. The study concluded that if a patient was pessimistic and believed that nothing would change, no matter what action she took, she is unlikely to read the information or understand it. This is particularly important with regard to personal health because sustained change is only possible if you accept that your personal behaviors are essential to the process. *You* control your health destiny.

Third, pessimists are more likely to have worse health because the number of perceived negative events that we experience in life is correlated with the number of medical illnesses we experience. Compelling medical evidence suggests that perceiving life events as negative is associated with diminished immune function. Laboratory assessments demonstrate a rise in the stress hormone cortisol at the time of life stressors such as job loss, divorce, the death of a spouse, or a family move.

These levels fall after the event, and it is not uncommon for a person to experience the illness of a common cold when those levels fall. I remember being in medical school, studying around the clock for examinations. I was so relieved to complete the tests, and I always developed the sniffles the week afterward.

I emphasize the term "perceived negative event" because what is described as a negative experience is in the eye of the beholder–how we explain the event. (Remember the exercise from Spoke Seven.) In his mind, Tiger Woods, while walking up the fairway in the midst of a sudden death tiebreaker, is having the competitive time of his life. If I offered most people the opportunity to complete a challenging task in front of millions of viewers, with the understanding that if they failed, they would be publicly and endlessly criticized, most would feel overwhelming pressure. They would likely say, "thanks, but no thanks." Yet top athletes face this pressure all the time and experience it as a positive motivation to succeed. The bottom line is that *perceived negative events* and stress are frequently related to depressed immune function and consequent illness.

This cycle is actually repetitive because pessimists are more likely to have negative events due to perceiving life's experiences from a passive perspective of learned helplessness and lack of control. Furthermore, they are less likely to take preventative and necessary steps (like going to the doctor or getting screening) to avoid negative events such as illness. After a bad event like a medical illness, they are less likely to take steps to improve their situation because of their learned helplessness. This leads to a greater number of lifetime negative events and resultant poor health. Additionally, the presence of a chronic medical condition, in general, is anxiety-provoking. Medications, tests, and periodic physician check-ups all serve as constant reminders that you have an ongoing problem.

This tells us how explanatory or attributional style determines your level of optimism. There are three critical factors in what you tell yourself about an event:

❖ Permanent versus temporary: Optimists explain and perceive positive circumstances in a permanent context and negative circumstances in a temporary context.

❖ Pervasive versus nonpervasive or global versus local: Optimists explain positive circumstances as pervasive or global and negative ones as nonpervasive or local.

❖ Internal versus external: Optimists explain positive outcomes in a personal attributional style and negative in a less personal style.

LEVEL OF OPTIMISM QUIZ

1.) You get hired for a job, even though the other applicants were extremely qualified. You think:
    a.) "I must be more qualified than I gave myself credit for!"
    b.) "I must have interviewed really well."

2.) Your child is named "Student of the Month." You think:
    a.) "Wow! My child is a really hard worker."
    b.) " Wow! My child is really lucky to get this honor."

3.) You find a dollar on the street. You think:
    a.) "Hey! How lucky!"
    b.) "Hey, I'm pretty observant!"

4.) You're trying to figure out a new computer program. After hours of work, it still eludes you. You think:
    a.) "Wow, technology has become so complicated! It'll take me a little longer to finally get this."
    b.) "I'm just not 'wired' to understand computers! I'm going to fall behind, but what can I do ?"

5.) You get an "A" on an exam. You think:
    a.) "Wow! I'm smart!"
    b.) "Wow! I was prepared!"

6.) Someone flips you off in traffic. You think:
    a.) "People are so rude!"
    b.) " That person must be having a bad day."

7.) You've planned a party in the park, but it rains on party day. You think:
    a.) "I should have planned better. I'm not really good with parties."
    b.) "Well, this is unlucky! My next party will by much more successful."

8.) You get a speeding ticket, and you realize you forget your wallet at home. You think:
    a.) "This must not be my day!"
    b.) "I am so unlucky!"

9.) You miss a flight and have to wait for another one. You think:
   a.) "If only there wasn't so much traffic! I guess I'll make the next flight."
   b.) "I should have planned better. I'm always late, and I knew this would happen."

10.) You find you don't have the money to pay all your bills at the end of the month. You think:
   a.) "It's been a slow month for business. Things will pick up next month."
   b.) "I'm not good at managing money. This is a serious problem."

11.) You've been working hard at dieting, and you lose ten pounds. You think:
   a.) "This diet really works! I hope I can lose more."
   b.) "My hard work is paying off! I'll be at my target weight in no time!"

12.) You meet an important business contact at a party. You think:
   a.) "Lucky me! I was in the right place at the right time."
   b.) "I was smart enough to come to this party tonight."

13.) You start a new workout program and are really sore the next day. You think:
   a.) "Wow, I must be out of shape!"
   b.) "Wow, I worked hard yesterday!"

Optimistic Answers:

1.) (a)
2.) (a)
3.) (b)
4.) (a)
5.) (a)
6.) (b)
7.) (b)
8.) (a)
9.) (a)
10.) (a)
11.) (b)
12.) (b)
13.) (b)

Optimists explain positive events as having happened because of themselves (internal attribution). They also see the positive events as evidence that more positive things will happen in the future (stability) and in other areas of their lives (global). Conversely, they see negative events as not their fault (external attribution). They also see them as flukes (isolated) that have nothing to do with other areas of their lives or future events (locality).

Pessimists think in the opposite way. They believe that they themselves cause negative events (internal attribution). They believe that one mistake means that more will come (stability) and that mistakes in other areas of life are inevitable (global), because they themselves are the cause. They see positive events as flukes (locality) that are caused by factors outside their control (external) and probably won't happen again (instability).

A pessimist would see a promotion as a lucky event that probably won't happen again and may even worry that he'll now be under more scrutiny. He would probably explain being passed over for promotion as due to his not having enough skills. He'd therefore expect to be passed over again.

In some circumstances, a pessimist's judgment is correct, and an action results in a poor outcome: failure. Sometimes, both pessimists and optimists fail. Yet interestingly, a pessimist will have a longer state of helplessness as a response to the same setback; that is, the failure will more profoundly and for a longer period of time paralyze a pessimist and prevent him from moving forward.

Now that you've had some experience in understanding the differences in the way that optimists and pessimists view life events, see if you can identify the different factors (internal versus external, stable versus isolated, global versus local) at work in the below positive and negative situations. Circle your optimistic thought and visit our Website for the answers.

OPTIMISTIC THOUGHT OR PESSIMISTIC THOUGHT?

1.) The project you are in charge of is a great success. You think:
   a.) "I kept a close watch over everyone's work."
   b.) "Everyone devoted a lot of time and energy to it."

2.) You get lost driving to a friend's house. You think:
   a.) "I missed a turn."
   b.) "My friend gave me bad directions."

3. Your spouse/partner/boyfriend/girlfriend surprises you with a gift. You think:
   a.) "He/she just got a raise at work."
   b.) "I took him/her out to a special dinner the night before."

4.) You forget your spouse's/partner's/boyfriend's/girlfriend's birthday. You think:
   a.) "I'm not good at remembering birthdays."
   b.) "I was preoccupied with other things."

5.) You get a flower from an admirer. You think:
   a.) "I am attractive to him/her."
   b.) "I am a popular person."

6.). You run for a community office position and win. You think:
   a.) "I devoted a lot of time and energy to campaigning."
   b.) "I work very hard at everything I do."

7.) You miss an important engagement. You think:
   a.) "Sometimes my memory fails me."
   b.) "I sometimes forget to check my appointment book."

8.) You run for a community office and lose. You think:
   a.) "I didn't campaign hard enough."
   b.) "The person who won knew more people."

9.) You host a successful dinner. You think:
   a.) "I was particularly charming that night."
   b.) "I am a good host."

10.) You gain weight over the holidays and can't lose it. You think:
   a.) "Diets don't work in the long run."
   b.) "The diet I tried didn't work."

11.) Your stocks make you a lot of money. You think:
   a.) "My broker decided to take on something new."
   b.) "My broker is a top-notch investor."

12.) You win an athletic contest. You think:
   a.) "I was feeling unbeatable."
   b.) "I train hard."

13.) You fail an important examination. You think:
   a.) "I wasn't as smart as the other people taking the exam."
   b.) "I didn't prepare for it well."

14.) You lose a sporting event for which you have been training for a long time. You think:
   a.) "I'm not very athletic."
   b.) "I'm not good at that sport."

15.) You lose your temper with a friend. You think:
   a.) "He/she is always nagging me."
   b.) "He/she was in a hostile mood."

16.) You are penalized for not returning your income tax forms on time. You think:
   a.) "I always put off doing my taxes."
   b.) "I was lazy about getting my taxes done this year."

17.) A game show host picks you out of the audience to participate in the show. You think:
   a.) "I was sitting in the right seat."
   b.) "I looked the most enthusiastic."

18.) You save a person from choking to death. You think:
   a.) "I know a technique to stop someone from choking."
   b.) "I know what to do in a crisis situation."

SOCIAL SUPPORTS

The final connection between pessimism and poor health relates to social supports. Studies suggest that the optimistic personality may be characterized by a greater number of friends and a social support network. Sincere friendship and genuine love seem to be important to our health. Maybe it is because a healthy social network of support provides us with an outlet to diffuse some of the stressors of life and perhaps avoid some of the subsequent physiologic insult that follows that perceived stress. Many of us have called our spouse or a good friend to unload, only to feel "less stressed" after talking it over, even though the situation has not changed. Studies also show that married couples tend to have a lower incidence of depression than their single counterparts.

The isolation caused by the lack of a consistent social network may cause an in ability to ward off illness. Patients with illness who isolate themselves tend to develop worse illness. Look no further than a modern hospital cancer ward that emphasizes connecting through support groups. The human connection that occurs when people open their hearts to others does seem to have an important role in health.

DRAWBACKS AND USES OF PESSIMISM

Pessimism, then, can have many detrimental effects on our life achievements, personal and family success, and our ability to achieve Optimal Health.

❖ Pessimists are more likely to develop a greater number of episodes of depression; their episodes are more likely to be prolonged.

❖ When faced with failure following an attempt to reach a goal, pessimists are more likely to develop inertia and assume a passive position.

❖ Pessimists are more likely to describe their emotional states of mind and their lives in relatively negative terms like blue, anxious, and stress-filled.

❖ Pessimism frequently results in unnecessary failure. It is self-fulfilling. Pessimists are less likely to take risks or put themselves in positions to succeed because of their passivity. When they execute an action to achieve a goal, if their first attempt is met with resistance and failure, pessimists are more likely to cease trying, even when, by outside assessment, the goal is achievable. This lack of perseverance is the hallmark of pessimists.

❖ Pessimism is associated with poor health and increased susceptibility to infection and disease.

But pessimism can't be all bad. To statements such as the above, a student of human development should rightfully counter: So where did this pessimistic personality characteristic come from? Most physical and behavioral characteristics originated as helpful behavioral habits that in some way facilitated survival and so were evolutionarily selected for. Pessimism—what some might refer to as caution—does have an important benefit in human survival. In a prehistoric world fraught with environmental dangers like animal predators, human adversaries, and natural disasters, caution clearly served as an evolutionary benefit for human survival. One can only imagine what happened to a tribal leader who recklessly led his family into nighttime travel across dangerous territory.

Thus, pessimists do excel in one area: the ability to view reality in a more conservative light. Sometimes, this pessimism and caution are beneficial. For example, a commercial building safety inspector in a metropolitan area like Manhattan has the challenging task of inspecting new skyscrapers for structural integrity. In the interest of public safety, a cautious personality quality that drives this individual's decisions is essential to effectively performing this job—and keeping us safe. I don't think we would want this person to throw caution to the wind when interpreting and enforcing building safety codes.

Our pessimistic voice does play a valuable role in a selected part of our daily decision-making processes. It can prevent us from embarking on some foolhardy, impulsive, poorly conceived endeavor toward which we might be occasionally tempted. I assert that we must have an appropriate balance and an appreciation for the precise situations in our lives in which pessimism might be advantageous.

But while the advocate of a pessimistic approach to life suggests that an optimist ignores the reality of a situation by burying her head in the sand to protect herself from reality, optimism does not propose to ignore reality. Instead, optimists appreci-ate the facts without attaching a negative emotional tag to the event or the outcome. They explain the facts of a negative event or outcome in a less personal, less tempo-rary fashion and attribute them less to their overall life circumstances.

OPTIMISM AND OPTIMAL HEALTH

As you can hopefully see, the benefits of an optimistic personality are limitless and can affect multiple facets of your life and relationships, including with your children, spouse, colleagues, and friends. Optimism is a valuable trait and a cherished gift to learn, develop, and share with others. The ability to develop an optimistic personality of thinking by fine-tuning your explanatory pattern to avoid temporary helplessness is essential to making and sustaining change in your life.

This includes your health. As Dr. Patel and I set out to create the Optimal Health Program, we knew it was important to have a single, essential component that pro-moted and in some plausible way explained this unique relationship between the mind and improved health. Optimism may be this component, along with balance and moderation. How important is developing such an explanatory style and optimistic personality to your health? Your explanatory style largely influences your health, lon-gevity, chronic stress levels, resistance to infection and perhaps cancer, and your over-all well-being and life achievements. When I first wrote this, I thought, "That sounds somewhat over-reaching; is that an exaggeration?" No, it's not. We have already dis-cussed the direct effect that optimism has on individual health. Perceived stress and other environmental stimuli prompt parts of our brains to release or inhibit neuro-hormonal modulators like cortisol, endorphins, and adrenaline. From a physiological standpoint, it is not difficult to connect the dots to describe the route by which our environment influences our behavior.

The global benefit to your life and the changes in your day-to-day outlook when you develop optimism are immeasurable. Our lives will always be filled with happiness and sorrow, elation and grief. Disasters will continue, with or without the tool of opti-mism. Optimism is not a short-term investment. If I go to Las Vegas with an optimistic belief that I will beat the house and walk away with a windfall, optimism may fail me in this short-term application. This is just like applying the concepts of your Personal Wellness Wheel™; if you eat better, get your labs checked, and exercise and medi-tate regularly, you may feel better temporarily. But without a long-term investment, you will not reach Optimal Health. However, if you alter your explanatory pattern and practices and apply these concepts in the context of your daily life experiences and to the principles of Optimal Health, I unequivocally assert that over time and at the final bell of life, you will have navigated life's gauntlet most effectively.

BUILDING SPOKE EIGHT
OF YOUR PERSONAL WELLNESS WHEEL™

❑ Decide *why* you want to work toward Optimal Health. Be as specific and as concrete as possible; consider all aspects of your life (your family, your work, your hobbies, etc.)

   ❖ What are your long-term goals?

   ❖ Why is developing your Personal Wellness Wheel™ beneficial to you?

❑ Explore the neuro-associations behind your thoughts about achieving Optimal Health and undertaking this eight-spoke program.

❖ What positive associations do you have regarding working toward Optimal Health? Write yourself reminders of these reasons and place them where you might see them, for example, near the refrigerator, near your clothes closet, in your planner.

❖ What negative associations do you have regarding toward Optimal Health? Where did they come from? How might you reframe them?

❑ Complete the optimism/pessimism quiz on pages 157 through 159; identify the factors at work in the thinking. Visit www.optimalhealthtoday.com to see the answers.

❑ Practice optimism in your life. Work at reframing the way you view events or explain them to yourself. If you find patterns in your life, you may want to write reminders to yourself to think optimistically.

   ❖ When something negative happens, remind yourself that it is temporary and will pass. Remind yourself of the good things in your life, that this event is just a small piece of your life overall, and that making mistakes is part of being human. If you do have a setback or fail, give yourself time to recover and then try again!

   ❖ When something positive happens, see it as a sign of good things yet to come. Did it happen due to your hard work, persistence, or character? If so, congratulate yourself!

❑ Find and associate with people who will help you work toward Optimal Health. Ask for help when you need it; this is especially important when you face challenges in striving toward Optimal Health. Many people and resources are ready and willing to assist you.

Most importantly, remember that
YOU are in control of your own health!
Each day is a chance to look good, feel great, and live better!

APPENDIX

CONTENTS:
* resources for Optimal Health
* Holmes-Rahe
life stress inventory
* bibliography

RESOURCES FOR OPTIMAL HEALTH

Below are resources to help you reach your goal of Optimal Health and continue building and maintaining your Personal Wellness Wheel™. Please also visit www.optimalhealthtoday.com to find a comprehensive guide to each spoke of the Personal Wellness Wheel™, as well as videos, podcasts, blogs, and a frequently updated list of Optimal Health Resources and Providers. Additionally, you can join the Optimal Health Forum to post your comments and exchange ideas with Dr. Patel and other informed members of the wellness community or sign up for the Institute for Optimal Health's monthly e-newsletter.

CHAPTERS 1 AND 2: PRO-ACTIVE, HEALTHY LIVING, AGE MANAGEMENT, AND INTEGRATIVE MEDICINE

Telephone Service:
Cancer Information Service (a program of the National Cancer Institute) 1-800-4-CANCER

Magazines and Websites about Healthy Living and Aging:
Healthy Aging (for physicians): www.healthy-aging.advanceweb.com
Healthy Living: www.freedompressonline.com
International Antiaging Magazine: www.antiaging-magazine.com
Life Extension: www.lef.org

Books:
Deepak Chopra, MD, *Ageless Body, Timeless Mind: The Quantum Alternative to Growing Old*. New York: Harmony Books, 1993.

Deepak Chopra, MD, *Perfect Health: The Complete Mind/Body Guide*. New York: Harmony Books, 1991.

Michael F. Roizen, MD, *The RealAge Makeover: Take Years Off Your Looks and Add Them to Your Life*. New York: HarperCollins, 2004.

Stephen T. Sinatra, *The Sinatra Solution: Metabolic Cardiology*. North Bergen, NJ: Basic Health Publications, 2005.

John H. K. Vogel and Mitchell W. Krucoff, eds. *Integrative Cardiology: Complementary and Alternative Medicine for the Heart.* New York: McGraw-Hill Medical, 2007.

Andrew Weil, MD, *Eight Weeks to Optimum Health: A Proven Program for Taking Full Advantage of Your Body's Natural Healing Power,* rev. ed. New York: Knopf, 2006.

<u>*Websites for General Medical Information:*</u>
Information about acupuncture: www.acupuncture.com
Information about Aruyveda: www.aruyveda.com
The Cancer Cure Coalition for the latest prevention and treatment of cancers:
www.cancercurecoalition.org
The Centers for Disease Control and Prevention, population-based health statistics
and programs: www.cdc.gov
The Green Guide (environmentally friendly green living): www.thegreenguide.com
Mayo Clinic information about common diseases and traditional medical treatments:
www.mayoclinic.com
Information about general medical conditions: www.familydoctor.org
National Center for Complementary and Alternative Medicine: www.nccam.nih.gov

CHAPTER 3: NUTRITION

<u>*Books:*</u>

Dr. Jennie Brand-Miller et al., *The New Glucose Revolution for Diabetes: The Definitive Guide to Managing Diabetes and Prediabetes Using the Glycemic Index.* New York: Avalon, 2007.

T. Colin Campbell, *The China Study: The Most Comprehensive Study of Nutrition Ever Conducted and the Starting Implications for Diet, Weight Loss and Long-Term Health.* Dallas, TX: BenBella Books, 2005.

Joshua Rosenthal, *Integrative Nutrition: Feed Your Hunger for Health and Happiness,* 2nd ed. New York: Integrative Nutrition Pub, 2008.

Gary Taubes, *Good Calories, Bad Calories: Challenging the Conventional Wisdom on Diet, Weight Control, and Disease.* New York: Knopf, 2007.

<u>*Websites:*</u>
Information about the glycemic index and glycemic load: www.glycemicindex.com
Learn what is in your food: www.labelwatch.com
The Organic Center (dedicated to the benefits of organic products and farming):
www.organiccenter.org

CHAPTER 4: EXERCISE

Book:

Phil Campbell, *Ready, Set, Go! Synergy Fitness.* New York: Fitness Publishers, 2001.

Websites for Finding a Personal Trainer:

The National Strength and Conditioning Association: www.nsca-lift.org

The American Council on Exercise: www.acefitness.org

The American College of Sports Medicine: www.acsm.org

CHAPTER 5: HORMONE OPTIMIZATION

Books:

Aaron E. Katz, MD, *Dr. Katz's Guide to Prostate Health: From Conventional to Holistic Therapies.* Topanga, CA: Freedom Press, 2006.

Ronald Klatz, MD, *Grow Young with HGH: The Amazing Medically Proven Plan to Reverse Aging.* New York: HarperCollins Publishers, 2007.

Christiane Northrup, MD, *The Wisdom of Menopause: Creating Physical and Emotional Health and Healing During the Change.* New York: Bantam Books, 2006.

Suzanne Somers, *Ageless: The Naked Truth About Bioidentical Hormones.* New York: Crown Publishers, 2006.

Websites:

General information on breast cancer: www.Breastcancer.org

Comprehensive information on cancer from the National Cancer Institute: www.cancer.gov

Information on menopausal hormone therapy, National Institutes of Health:
www.nih.gov/PHTindex.htm

National Ovarian Cancer Coalition: www.ovarian.org

Prostatitis Foundation: www.prostatitis.org

CHAPTER 6: AGELESS SKIN

Books:

Leslie Baumann, MD, *The Skin Type Solution.* New York: Bantam Books, 2007.

Nicholas Perricone, MD, *The Wrinkle Cure: Unlock the Power of Cosmeceuticals for Supple, Youthful Skin.* Emmaus, PA: Rodale, 2000.

Websites:

Site dedicated to the unique needs of African-American skin: www.blackskincareonline.com

American Academy of Dermatology (skin topics from A-Z): www.aad.org/dermaz

American Society of Plastic Surgeons information: www.plasticsurgery.org

CHAPTER 7: STRESS MANAGEMENT THROUGH MEDITATION AND MINDFULNESS

Books:

Thich Nhat Hahn, *The Miracle of Mindfulness: A Manual of Meditation*. Boston: Beacon Press, 1987

Geshe Kelsang Gyatso, *The New Meditation Handbook: Meditations to Make Our Life Happy and Meaningful*, 4th ed. Glen Spey, NY: Tharpa Publications, 1993.

Websites:

Modern meditation CD: www.kathleenohara.com

Mindfulness meditation tapes and CDs by Dr. Jon Kabat-Zinn: www.mindfulnessstapes.com

CHAPTER 8: STRATEGIES FOR SUCCESS

Books:

Martin E. P. Seligman, *Learned Optimism: How to Change Your Mind and Your Life*. New York: Vintage Books, 2006.

Anthony Robbins, *Awaken the Giant Within: How to Take Immediate Control of Your Mental, Emotional, Physical & Financial Destiny!* New York: Simon & Schuster, 1992.

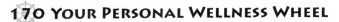

HOLMES-RAHE LIFE STRESSOR INVENTORY

Circle the stressors you have had in the past six months.

Stressor	Score
Death of spouse	100
Divorce	75
Marital separation	65
Jail term	63
Death of a close family	63
Personal injury or illness	53
Marriage	50
Fired from job	47
Marital reconciliation	45
Retirement	45
Change in family member's health	44
Pregnancy	40
Sexual difficulties	39
Addition to the family	39
Business readjustment	39
Change in financial status	38
Death of close friend	37
Career change	36
Change in marital arguments	35
Mortgage or loan over $100,000	35

Foreclosure of mortgage or loan	30
Change in work responsibilities	29
Son or daughter leaving home	29
Trouble with in-laws	29
Outstanding personal achievement	29
Spouse begins or ceases work	26
Starting or finishing school	26
Change in living conditions	25
Revision of personal habits	23
Trouble with boss	23
Change in work hours/conditions	20
Change in residence	20
Change in school	20
Change in recreational habits	19
Change in church or social activities	18
Change in number of family gatherings	15
Change in eating habits	15
Vacation	13
Christmas season	12
Minor violation with the law	11

Add up your score. If it is greater than 150, your stress is high. You must do something to deal with this stress before it affects your health. If it has already impacted your health, dealing with the stress will help improve your health.

BIBLIOGRAPHY

Chapter One:
A Pro-Active Health Approach: Preventing Disease

Centers for Disease Control and Prevention (CDC). (2002). "Annual Smoking-Attributable Mortality, Years of Potential Life Lose and Productivity-US 1997-2001." *Morbidity and Mortality Weekly Report*, Vol. 51, No. 12, 12 April 2002, pp. 300-303.

CDC. (2004). *The Health Consequences of Smoking: A Report of the Surgeon General.* Washington, DC: US Department of Health and Human Services.

CDC. (2007). "Mortality Rates in the U.S." Washington, DC: US Department of Health and Human Services.

Silagy, C. (2008). "Nicotine Replacement Therapy for Smoking Cessation." *Cochrane Database of Systemic Reviews*, 23 January, 2008: (1)CD000146.

Chapter Five:
Hormone Optimization:
Restoring Your Body's Balance

Araujo, A. (2007). "Prevalence of Symptomatic Androgen Deficiency in Men." *The Journal of Clinical Endocrinology and Metabolism*, Vol. 92, No. 11, pp. 4241-4247.

Becker, K. et al. (2001). *Principles for Endocrinology and Metabolism*. Philadelphia: Lippincott, Williams, and Wilcott.

Bolour, S. (2005). "Testosterone Therapy in Women: A Review." *International Journal of Impotence Research*, Vol. 17, Sept-Oct 2005, pp. 399-408.

Carrero, J. (2007). "Clinical and Biological Implications of Low Thyroid Hormones in Euthyroid Patients with Chronic Kidney Disease." *Journal of Internal Medicine*, Vol. 262, No. 6, December 2007, pp. 690-701.

CDC. (2006). "Prostate Cancer Screening: A Decision Guide for African Americans." Washington DC: Division of Cancer Prevention and Control, National Center for Chronic Disease Prevention and Health Promotion.

Chung, J. (2004). "Intrinsic Aging and Photoaging Pathophysiology." In Rigel, *Photoaging* (p. 8). New York: Marcel Dekker, Inc.

Cobin, R. M. (2006). "American Association of Clinical Endocrinologists Medical Guidelines for Clinical Practice for the Diagnosis and Treatment of Menopause." *Endocrinology Practice*, Vol. 12, No. 3, July 2006, pp. 315-337.

Cutson, T. M. (2006). "Managing Menopause." *American Family Physician*, Vol. 61, 3 March 2006, pp. 1391-40.

Eedy, D. (2006). "Updates from the British Association of Dermatologists." *British Journal of Dermatology*, Vol. 154, No. 6, June 2006, pp. 1028-1045.

Feldmen, H. (2002). "Age Trends in the Level of Serum Testosterone and Other Hormones in Middle Aged Men." *Journal of Clinical Endocrinology & Metabolism*, Vol. 87, No. 2, February 2002, pp. 589-598.

Gurnell, E. (2001). "DHEA: A Mini Review." *European Journal of Endocrinology*, Vol. 145, Issue 2, April 2001, pp. 103-106.

Helfand, M. (2004). "Screening for Subclinical Thyroid Dysfunction in Non Pregnant Adults." *Annals of Internal Medicine*, Vol. 140, Issue 2, January 2004, pp. 128-141.

Hornum, M. (1997). "Exercise Induced Changes in Circulating Growth Factors with Cyclic Variation in Estradiol in Women." *Journal of Applied Physiology*, Vol. 82, No. 6, June 1997, pp. 1946-1951.

Hulley, S. (1998). "Randomized Trial of Estrogen Plus Progestin for Secondary Prevention of Coronary Artery Disease in Post Menopausal Women." *Journal of the American Medical Association*, Vol. 280, No. 7, 19 August 1998, pp. 605-613.

Iervasi, G. (2003). "Low T3–A Strong Prognostic Indicator of Death in Patients with Heart Disease." *Circulation*, Vol. 107, Issue 5, February 2003, pp. 708-713.

Iervasi, G. (2007). "Association between Increased Mortality and Mild Thyroid Dysfunction in Cardiac Patients." *Archives of Internal Medicine*, Vol. 167, No. 14, 23 July 2007, pp. 1526-1532.

International Menopause Society, adapted from. (2008). "Hormone Replacement Therapy is Safe for Women Entering Menopause, Summit Concludes." *Science Daily*, 21 May 2008. Available at www.sciencedaily.com/releases/2008/05/080520090430.htm

Jankowski, C. (2006). "Effects of DHEA Therapy on Bone Mineral Density in Older Adults." *Journal of Clinical Endocrinology and Metabolism*, Vol. 91, issue 8, August 2006, pp. 2986-2993.

Kalyani, R. (2007). "Male Hypogonadism in Systemic Disease." *Endocrinology and Metabolism Clinics in North America*, Vol. 36, Issue 2, 2 June 2007, pp. 333-348.

Liverman, C. (2004). *Testosterone and Clinical Research Directions*. Washington DC: National Academies Press.

Miller, K. (2001). "Androgen Deficiency in Women." *Journal of Clinical Endocrinology & Metabolism*, Vol. 91, Issue 5, May 2006, pp. 2395-2401.

Miller, K. (2006). "Effects of Testosterone Replacement in Androgen-Deficient Women with Hypopituitarism: A Randomized, Double-Blind, Placebo-Controlled Study." *Journal of Clinical Endocrinology & Metabolism*, Vol. 91, Issue 5, May 2006, pp. 1683-1690.

Molitich, M. (2006). "Evaluation and Treatment of Adult Growth Hormone Deficiency: An Endocrine Society Clinical Practice Guideline." *Journal of Clinical Endocrinology & Metabolism*, Vol. 91, Issue 5, May 2006, pp. 1621-1634.

Morales, A. (2002). "Androgen Deficiency in the Aging Male: Who, When and How to Investigate and Treat." *Urologic Clinics of North America*, Vol. 9, No. 4, Nov. 2002, pp. 975-982.

NAMS. (2005). "The Role of Testosterone Therapy in Post Menopausal Women." *Menopause*, Vol. 12, No. 5, Nov/Dec 2005, pp. 496-511.

National Institutes of Health. (2007). *Osteoporosis Overview*. Washington DC: National Resource Center.

Pepping, J. (2000). "DHEA–Dihydroepiandrosterone." *American Journal of Health System Pharmacy*, Vol. 57, No. 22, Nov. 2002, pp. 2048-2056.

Pines, A. (2008). "HRT in Early Menopause: Scientific Evidence and Common Perceptions," written as a consensus report at the International Menopause Society, Zurich, Switzerland, March 2008.

Pompei, P. (2006). *Geriatrics Review Syllabus: A Core Curriculum in Geriatric Medicine*. Boston: Blackwell Publishing.

Rodondi, N. (2006). "Subclinical Hypothyroid Disease and the Risk for Coronary Heart Disease: A Meta-analysis." *American Journal of Medicine*, Vol. 119, Issue 7, July 2006, pp. 541-551.

Rousseau, J. (2002). "Risks and Benefits of Estrogen Plus Progestin in Healthy Postmenopausal Women." *Journal of American Medical Association*, pp. 321-333.

Sarrell, P. (1999). "Psychosocial Effects of Menopause: Role of Androgens." *Journal of Obstetrics and Gynecology*, Vol. 180, supplement, March 1999, pp. 319-324.

Schmidt, P. (2005). "DHEA as Monotherapy in Midlife Onset Major and Minor Depression." *Archives of General Psychiatry*, Vol. 62, No. 2, pp. 154-162.

Sherwin, B. (1996). "Estrogen, the Brain, and Memory." *Menopause: The Journal of the North American Menopause Society*, Vol. 3, No. 2, pp. 97-105.

Sonntag, W. (1995). "Moderate Caloric Restriction Alters the Subcellular Distribution of Somatostatin mRNA and Increases Growth Hormone Pulse Amplitude in Aged Animals." *Neuroendocrinology*, Vol. 68, No. 1, pp. 601-608.

Surks, M. (2004). "Subclinical Thyroid Disease: Scientific Review and Guidelines for Diagnosis and Management." *Journal of the American Medical Association*, Vol. 291, No. 2, July 2004, pp. 228-238.

Tamimi, R. (2006). "Combined Estrogen and Testosterone Use and Risk of Breast Cancer in Post Menopausal Women." *Archives of Internal Medicine*, Vol. 166, No. 14, July 2006, pp. 1483-1489.

Vahl, N. (1996). Abdominal Adiposity and Physical Fitness are Major Determinants of the Age Associated Decline in Stimulated GH Secretion in Healthy Adults. *Journal of Clinical Endocrinology and Metabolism*, Vol. 81, Issue 6, June 1996, pp. 2209-2215.

Wilson, G. (2005). "Subclinical Thyroid Disease." *American Academy of Family Practice*, Vol. 72, No. 8, Oct. 2005, pp. 1517-1524.

INDEX

ABOUT THE AUTHOR

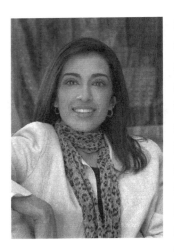

Dr. Seema Patel is the co-founder of The Institute for Optimal Health & Advanced Skincare. She is recognized for her groundbreaking concepts in aging and skincare. For years, aging and skincare have been perceived and managed as two distinct processes. Yet internal aging and skin appearance are clearly not distinct events. A renowned expert in laser cosmetic surgery, injectable skin treatments, and topical skincare regimens, Dr. Patel combines these with her extensive advanced training and specialized credentials in Age Management from The Cenegenics Medical Institute. Her innovative approach to combining age management strategies with the latest scientifically based approaches to skin care enables patients to "look good, feel great, and live better" at any age. Her extensive training and broad interests facilitate her skill in treating patients of all ages and skin tones with equal comfort.

Dr. Patel is a graduate of the University of Michigan and The Ohio State University College of Medicine. She completed a Master's in Public Health (with a concentration in Preventative Medicine and Health Policy) at the University of Michigan. She is a Fellow of the American Society of Lasers in Medicine and Surgery and a member of the Society of Dermatology Skin Care Specialists, the Medical Spa Society, the American Academy of Family Physicians, and the American Public Health Association. She was voted top Family Physician by *Consumer Reports* in 2006 and 2007 and is the recipient of many national academic honors and awards. Dr. Patel is an expert injector of Restylane®, Juvederm®, and Botox Cosmetic®. She has educated the public and other medical care providers about the rapid changes in the anti-aging and skincare markets.

Dr. Patel currently lives in Philadelphia, Pennsylvania, with her husband, Dr. Lee Kirksey, who wrote sections of *Your Guide to Optimal Health*. For fun, she has traveled extensively throughout the world, including Africa, Asia, Europe, and Latin America. She is fluent in three languages and is an avid runner who has completed the Chicago and New York City marathons and countless smaller distance runs. Dr. Patel had her first child in October 2007.

2445263